Treating Fearful Dental Patients

A PATIENT MANAGEMENT HANDBOOK

Treating Fearful Dental Patients
A PATIENT MANAGEMENT HANDBOOK

Peter Milgrom, D.D.S.
Associate Professor, Department of Community Dentistry
University of Washington School of Dentistry
Seattle, Washington

Philip Weinstein, Ph.D.
Associate Professor, Department of Community Dentistry
University of Washington School of Dentistry
Seattle, Washington

Ronald Kleinknecht, Ph.D.
Professor, Psychology Department
Western Washington University
Bellingham, Washington

Tracy Getz, M.S.
Lecturer, Department of Community Dentistry
University of Washington School of Dentistry
Seattle, Washington

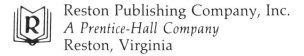
Reston Publishing Company, Inc.
A Prentice-Hall Company
Reston, Virginia

Library of Congress Cataloging in Publication Data

Main entry under title:

Treating fearful dental patients.

  Bibliography: p.
    1. Dentistry—Psychological aspects.   2. Fear.
3. Dentist and patient.   I. Milgrom, Peter. [DNLM:
1. Fear.   2. Patients—psychology.   3. Dental Care—
psychology.   4. Dentist-Patient Relations.   WU 61 T784]
RK53.T74   1985   617.6′0019   84-23726
ISBN 0-8359-7829-X

© 1985 by Reston Publishing Company, Inc.
A Prentice-Hall Company
Reston, Virginia 22090

10 9 8 7 6 5 4 3 2 1

Printed in the United States of America

Contents

Introduction

This book was conceived as a practical handbook for both students and practicing professionals, dentists, dental hygienists, and assistants. Our goal is to provide an understanding of the development and nature of dental fear, and to explain the fundamental skills necessary to successfully treat the fearful patient.

We are clinicians who are active in research and in the treatment of patients who are afraid of the dentist, and together we share 40 years of practice experience. We blend results from our research in this area with clinical insights in a way that they illustrate and enhance the usefulness of each. We have purposely attempted to walk the thin line between a scholarly presentation and an anecdotal breezy approach to create a readable, useful, but scientific text.

A question we are often asked is: Are your clinic patients really phobic, or are they merely fearful? Our response to this is another question. Is a patient who avoided dentistry for 15 years and comes in with a need for three endodontic treatments, two molars fractured to the gum line, and missing anteriors fearful or phobic? Definitions and categories are useful if they provide information relevant to the treatment strategies employed. It has been our experience that there is no practical difference between fearful and phobic.

Why bother to learn "special" skills to treat the fearful patient? There are three very apparent reasons.

The first involves the issue of "busyness." Studies indicate that less than one half of the American population goes to the dentist once a year. Studies have also shown that somewhere between 6 and 14 percent of the American population (14,000,000–34,000,000) avoid dentistry completely because of fear. It is estimated that another 20–30 percent dislike dentistry enough to be only occasional users. Fear is a very real barrier to seeking out dental services. In addition, if you reduce an individual's anxiety, you increase the probability that he will follow through on recommended treatment plans and will return for recall. We believe that the ability to recognize and successfully treat the anxious patient results in many new patients and fewer fear related cancellations and failures.

Secondly, learning to treat the fearful patient will reduce your own personal level of stress. Surveys have repeatedly shown that the most frustrating aspect of dental practice is working with the "difficult" patient. By learning skills to help you work with the fearful individual, you will reduce the stress of dental practice and the potential of professional burn-out.

Finally, there is the personal reward of helping a person overcome a difficult barrier. Long after we forget our finest technical accomplishments, we take satisfaction from being able to truly make a significant difference in another person's life.

This book is an attempt to pull together knowledge from many different areas of psychology and dentistry and apply it to the care of patients. All the answers have not been found nor even all the questions asked. We invite you to give us feedback regarding your reactions to the concepts and strategies presented, and use the reader response form on the following page.

READER FEEDBACK FORM

We have found the techniques and procedures described in this book to be helpful to our patients and have tried to convey these and the current research in fear treatment to you. However, we realize that we may not have included something for everyone or to meet every patient that you might see in your practice. Also we may not have described our techniques in a fashion that allowed you to make direct applications to your patients.

To assist us in making future editions of this book more useful to the provider, we would greatly appreciate your comments to the questions below. These questions are designed for you to tell us what features and areas of this book you found useful and those which were not helpful or useful. Please address your reponses to:

Dr. Peter Milgrom
University of Washington
Dental Fears Research Clinic
Seattle, Washington 98195

1. Please describe those features of the book that you found most useful in understanding and treating fearful patients.

_____

_____

_____

_____

2. Note those features or areas of the book that were not useful, were confusing, or that did not seem to work for you.

_____

_____

_____

_____

3. Describe any specific changes to enhance the book's clinical usefulness.

_____

_____

_____

4. Describe any cases in which you were able to successfully apply the procedures described to reduce patient's fears. Please include patient characteristics and the procedures you used.

_____

_____

_____

5. Describe any cases in which you were unable to apply these techniques. Where and how did the book fail to give you what was needed? Please give patient details and what you tried that did not seem to work.

_____

_____

_____

6. Any other comments.

_____

_____

_____

7. Your name and address: (optional)

_____

_____

_____

ONE

The Problem of Fear in Dentistry

Joan is a 36-year-old, college educated mother of two children. Joan had avoided dentistry totally for the past six years. Not only did she not go herself, she could not even take her children to the pedodontist. At her husband's urging, she finally consented to go for an examination, but only if he made the appointment. Even though she was administered nitrous oxide, Joan experienced an intense fear reaction during the examination. Within minutes she was virtually soaked with perspiration and experienced shortness of breath, muscle tension, weakness in her knees, and nausea. She felt an overpowering desire to get out of the office, which she did with the examination only partially completed. Afterwards, she felt "humiliated, embarrassed and childish. My children can be braver than I was."

Intense fear is one of the most debilitating and agonizing human emotional experiences. It is also one of the most necessary and adaptive emotions. Fear is the motivating force that keeps us from dangers. Although the capacity to experience fear is an innate biological function, our responses of fear to certain objects and situations are largely acquired through our daily learning experiences. As children, we are taught that it is dangerous to play with fire, to play in the street, to talk to strangers, or to venture too far from home. Indeed, a large part of our early learning consists of learning to identify and to avoid potential threats to our well-being.

The development of fear responses to potentially threatening situations is normal, natural, and adaptive. However, the acquisition of fear responses to perceived threats can proceed in a seemingly non-rational and indiscriminant manner. That is, fear can become associated with a wide variety of environmental objects and situations. Some may pose actual serious threats and therefore appear "rational." Others may be clearly "irrational," while yet others may have some degree of rationality but the reaction appears out of proportion to the actual threat. However, it is important to realize that what determines an individual's reaction to a situation is *not* an outsider's view or judgment of the actual or potential threat.

Rather, it is the individual's own personal perception of the situation—which is based on his/her past experiences and current interpretation of the present situation.

Joan's earliest memory of dentistry was when she accompanied her mother to the dentist: "I remember waiting in the car. I could see my mother in the chair through a window. She was crying and the dentist was scolding her. I saw the dentist place a cloth over mother's head and face and leave the room. When mother returned to the car she was still crying and very upset."

A powerful and frightening message had been communicated to Joan: "The dentist hurt my mother and he could also hurt me." When Joan was later taken to this same dentist, he scolded her for being a "brat." Out of what she felt was self-defense, she bit his finger when he tried to examine her teeth. Later, she recalled a number of subsequent appointments with this dentist, all of which were reported to be very frightening and painful. These experiences fulfilled her negative expectations concerning dentistry which began with her earlier observation of her mother's experience.

This history of Joan's reactions and early experiences with dentistry is not uncommon among fearful patients. Although briefly described, it illustrates several points concerning dental fear which will be made repeatedly and described in greater detail throughout this book. First, in all other aspects of her life, Joan was an intelligent, stable, and responsible person. She was a good mother to her children, a good wife to her husband, maintained her household and a small farm, and had no other problems requiring psychological intervention. Her reaction to dentistry was the only area of her life with which she was unable to cope. This is true of the majority of fearful patients. Secondly, her seemingly irrational reaction, as viewed from the outside, became more understandable and "rational" after considering her early experiences and associations with dentists. From her experiences, she perceived dentistry as a threat to her well-being. The fear kept her from re-experiencing dentistry, an event that could have changed this perception. Also, if an assessment of her prior dental experiences had been conducted, she would have been spared the trauma and humiliation she experienced and treatment for her fear could have begun sooner.

Finally, through referral to one of us, her fear of dentistry was overcome in a very short time by applying the assessment and treatment procedures to be described in this book. Because she had avoided treatment for so long, she needed extensive restorative treatment. Within the six months following treatment for her fear, she made and kept five treatment appointments. Further, she felt proud of herself for having conquered her fear, for getting the needed dental treatment, and for finally being able to take her children to the pedodontist. This treatment was effective because a program was designed for her specific needs and allowed her to be carefully re-introduced to dentistry by a skillful and concerned dentist.

DEFINITIONS OF FEAR TERMINOLOGY

Thus far we have used the term *fear* without providing a definition. Although most people intuitively know what fear is, it is important to clarify more precisely what we mean by it, and how it differs from the related terms of *anxiety* and *phobia*.

Fear

Fear is an individual's emotional response to a perceived threat or danger. This response is composed of three related components: (1) an unpleasant cognitive state, such as the feeling that something terrible is going to happen; (2) physiologic changes, primarily involving activation of the sympathetic branch of the autonomic nervous system. Intense fear reactions will typically include tachycardia, profuse perspiration, respiration changes such as hyperventilation, muscle tension, gastrointestinal upset, and other physiologic signs of emotional arousal; and (3) overt behavioral movements, such as jitteriness, shakes, pacing, and attempts to escape or avoid the perceived threat.

This constellation of fear responses is called the "fight or flight" response (Cannon, 1929). The arousal of fear is seen as generally adaptive because it prepares and mobilizes the body to confront (fight) the threat or to escape from it (flight). We will discuss this fear response and its components in greater detail in Chapter 3.

Anxiety

Anxiety is frequently used to denote an emotional experience similar to fear as we have defined it. In fact, there are some writers who use the two terms as synonymous. However, we find it useful to differentiate between the two while recognizing that the responses are similar. We use the term anxiety to denote responses to situations in which the source of threat to the individual is ill-defined, ambiguous, or not immediately present. In other words, anxiety is used to denote reactions to non-immediate situations. For example, one who reacts emotionally to the anticipation of some *future* event would be said to experience "anticipatory anxiety." Accordingly, a person confronted on a dark street by a mugger, who experiences apprehension and increased heart rate and feels like running, would be said to be *fearful*. On the other hand, a person who, in the safety of his own home, senses a feeling of dread, whose heart races, and who begins to shake all over at the thought that next week he may confront a mugger, would be said to be experiencing anxiety. The major difference is the immediacy of the stimulus. A response to an immediate threat is fear.

In this book we will use the term *fear* when referring to a response at the dentist's office. *Anxiety* will be used to denote reactions in anticipation or at the thought of dentistry.

Phobia

Yet another term used to denote these same responses is phobia. Phobia is a special form of intense fear. The *Diagnostic and Statistical Manual* (DSM III, 1980) of the American Psychiatric Association defines phobia as a ". . . persistent and irrational fear of a specific object, activity or situation that results in a compelling desire to avoid the dread object, activity or situation (phobic stimulus). The fear is recognized by the individual as ex-

6

cessive or unreasonable in proportion to the actual dangerousness . . ." (APA, 1980, p. 225.)

This statement goes on to note that when the avoidance is of such proportion that it causes significant distress or interferes with one's social or role functioning, the reaction qualifies as a phobia.

Other characterizations of phobias include statements that they cannot be explained or reasoned away and that they are beyond voluntary control (Marks, 1969.) According to these criteria, Joan's reaction to having a dental exam would clearly qualify for the diagnosis of phobia.

As we will see, reactions to dentistry can come in all degrees of intensity and rationality. That is, some people have only mild apprehension, which causes little problem, while others may avoid even the thought or word "dentistry" at all cost.

AN APPROACH-AVOIDANCE CONCEPTUALIZATION FOR DETERMINING THE DEGREE OF PATIENT FEAR

In this section we describe a patient classification system that we have found useful in treatment. This classification system is based in part on the concepts of approach and avoidance tendencies originally described by Lewin (1931) and later explicated by Dollard and Miller (1950) from their research on the nature and effects of fear. Before describing the classifications, we will outline the concepts of the *approach-avoidance conflict*.

An approach-avoidance conflict exists when a person has two competing tendencies with respect to a single situation. That is, a person may want to attain a goal but at the same time avoid it. Relating this to dentistry, we can envision a person who knows he needs dental care and wants to have attractive, healthy teeth. In other words, the person is motivated to approach a dentist. At the same time, the person is fearful of going to the dentist and desires to avoid it. These two competing tendencies, one to approach and one to avoid, leave the person in a state of conflict. Miller and Dollard further found through their research that the two tendencies change in strength as the person in conflict moves closer to or further from the desired but feared situation. As one is further away in time or distance, the approach tendency is stronger than the avoidance tendency. But as one nears the feared situation, the avoidance tendency increases in strength more quickly than does the approach tendency. This situation is illustrated in Figure 1-1. The lines called *goal gradients* in this figure represent the different approach and avoidance tendencies. The slope of the gradient going from "close" to "far" from the goal is different for the two tendencies. When the person is far away from the goal, the approach tendency is higher or stronger than the avoidance. As he moves closer, he reaches a point where the two tendencies are of equal strength (where the gradients intersect). At this point, the person is torn by two equally strong tendencies. If the person were placed closer to the dentist's office, the avoidance tendency would be stronger, causing him to retreat. But as he got past the intersection, the approach tendency would be strongest. The person is caught between these competing response tendencies.

   This conceptualization can help explain a common occurrence seen among fearful patients and one that causes dentists and their staffs considerable problems: that of the patient cancelling or not appearing for appointments they have made. When the appointment is far off, say three

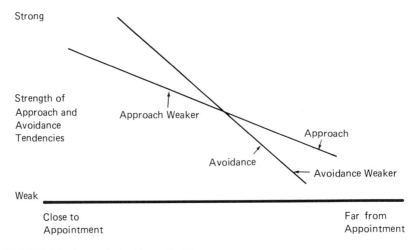

FIGURE 1-1. *Approach-Avoidance Conflict.*

8

weeks away, the approach tendency is stronger than the avoidance and the person is able to call for an appointment. It doesn't seem so bad at a distance. The person may have some anxiety, but the desire for needed dental care is stronger. As the time draws closer to the actual appointment, the avoidance tendency becomes stronger than the approach tendency. At this point, the anxiety becomes too strong to resist and the person does not "show." The result is that the dentist is frustrated because he has a vacancy in his schedule. The patient too may feel frustrated with himself for "being such a coward" and for not getting the dental care he needs and wants.

In order to break this cycle of approaching and avoiding, something must intervene to lower the avoidance gradient and/or to raise the approach gradient. For example, if a fearful person who has avoided and/or cancelled several prophylactic appointments due to fear develops a severe toothache, the pain may be enough to raise the approach gradient sufficiently to exceed the avoidance tendency. Or, a fearful patient may meet a dentist socially and find he or she to be a concerned and caring person, very different from his prior image of dentists. The changed attitude about dentists' concern for patients may be sufficient to lower the avoidance gradient. The subsequent chapters of this book are devoted to these goals: decreasing the fear and avoidance gradient and/or increasing the motivation or approach gradient. For now, let's turn to a classification system that describes some of the types of fearful patients seen in dental practice, using the approach-avoidance concepts.

The types of patients described here are presented mainly for illustrative purposes and should not be taken as a diagnostic system. However, practitioners who have dealt with fearful or apprehensive patients will be able to classify many of their patients using these categories.

The Apprehensive Patient

This classification encompasses the largest proportion of patients who experience some degree of dental fear. The term "apprehensive" is used to describe them because the fear experienced is relatively moderate and does not lead to avoidance or necessarily cause significant treatment

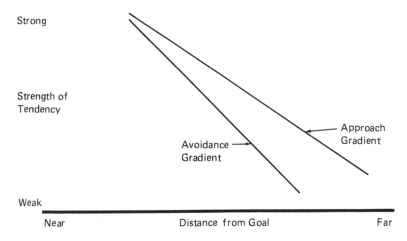

FIGURE 1-2. *Approach-Avoidance Gradient for the Apprehensive Patient.*

problems. The situation is graphically displayed in Figure 1-2. Using the approach-avoidance concepts, the approach gradient is higher than the avoidance gradient, allowing the person to appear at the office. However, by the time the patient arrives, the avoidance gradient comes very close to intersecting and the patient begins to experience some fear.

These patients will experience some discomfort both in anticipation of an appointment and while in the dental office. They may say to themselves, "I hope he doesn't find any cavities," or "I hope this is quick," or "Hope this won't hurt." Similar statements may be made to the dentist or assistant, but often with a nervous type of humor. This patient is little problem to the provider. He or she is generally cooperative and may successfully mask apprehension for fear of looking "childish." In fact, many patients within this category have successfully masked their fear to the extent that the dentist may have no idea that they are experiencing any discomfort. It is important to note here, however, that many such apprehensive patients may be potential phobic patients. If they experience sufficient pain or discomfort or believe that they have not been treated well, their fear may increase enough to raise their avoidance gradient. The result might be that they seek a new dentist who will be more attentive to their general comfort or avoid dentistry altogether. In later sections of this book we will discuss procedures for dental personnel to use to identify such patients.

"Goers but Haters"

Patients in this category also attend on a relatively regular basis but experience considerably more intense fear than the Apprehensive Patient. They may begin their worrying days in advance of their appointment. As the appointment day approaches, their approach and avoidance gradients come closer and closer to intersecting, as the fear rises (see Figure 1-3). However, once the appointment is set, they feel a strong obligation to follow through with it. This motivation keeps their approach gradient enough above their avoidance gradient to ensure that they appear at the office.

As can be seen in Figure 1-3, the approach avoidance gradients are not too different from those of the Apprehensive Patient. The main factor differentiating them is that the avoidance gradient is steeper. However, the

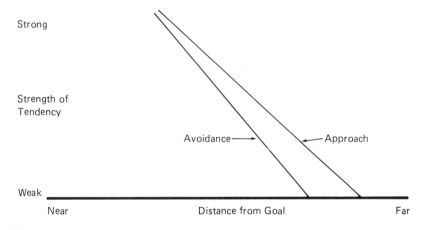

FIGURE 1-3. Approach-Avoidance Gradients for the "Goer but Hater."

approach gradient is also high because of a commitment to appear once an appointment has been made.

Once in the office, their fear level causes them considerable discomfort, and they are less able to hide or mask it. These patients may tell the dentist directly that they "hate dentistry," and cause problems for the dentist. Such patients who are visibly upset stop the dentist, frequently need to be told to "open wider," "to relax," etc. Further, this then causes considerable stress on the dentist, knowing that the patient is reacting to him or his treatment. Such patients require more time to treat and often cause the dentist to get behind schedule, further increasing the stress. The result is an unpleasant experience for both patient and dentist.

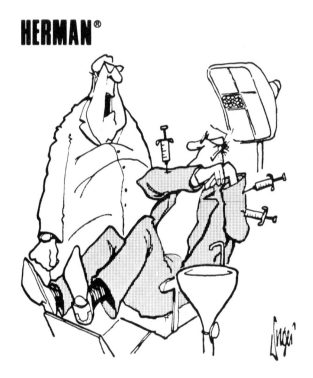

HERMAN®

"WILL YOU KEEP YOUR ARMS DOWN!"

Partial Avoiders

Patients classified as partial avoiders are similar in many respects to the "Goers but Haters." However, their fear causes them to put off making appointments for years at a time. If their fear is not treated, they are unlikely to become regular dental patients. In other words, their avoidance tendency is considerably stronger than their approach tendency, and they continue to avoid as long as possible (see Figure 1-4).

At some point, other factors intervene to raise the approach gradient, (as depicted by the dotted line in Figure 1-4). Typical factors motivating them to approach are urging by family members who may actually make the appointment or the occurrence of some dental problem that renders their discomfort greater than their fear.

The emotional suffering experienced is similar in intensity to that of the "Goer but Hater," but the anticipatory discomfort lasts longer. Because of the length of time between appointments, these patients may require rather extensive treatment. They require longer times to treat because of both the fear and neglect, further increasing their discomfort. Stress on the dentist is similar to that noted for the "Goer but Hater."

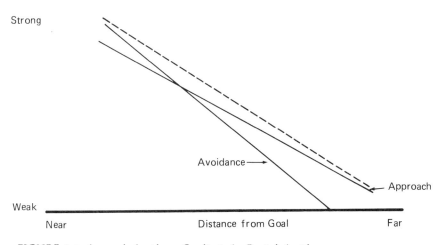

FIGURE 1-4. Approach-Avoidance Gradients for Partial Avoiders.

Total Avoiders

Total avoiders will rarely be seen in dental offices. They avoid dentistry at all costs. Their main contact with dentistry is through emergency clinics where they may appear in excruciating pain. Their avoidance gradient is well above their approach gradient and the two rarely intersect (see Figure 1-5).

Such patients will often tolerate very high levels of dental pain rather than submit themselves to even emergency dental care. The pain experienced from the dental problem far exceeds what they might experience at the hands of the dentist. The extreme avoidance, clearly irrational and interfering with daily functioning, qualifies as a phobia.

Persons with extreme dental phobias self-medicate. They use alcohol and/or other pain-killing drugs and not uncommonly will be under the influence when they appear at an emergency clinic. For most, they see the ultimate solution to their problems as having all their teeth extracted under general anesthesia. Treatment of patients presenting such intense fear and pain is exceedingly difficult. Unless treated for their fear, they are unlikely to return for subsequent appointments.

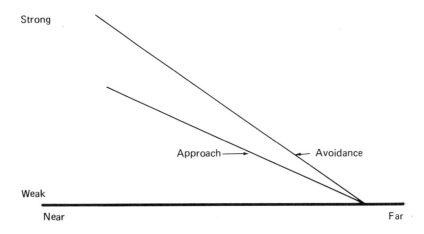

FIGURE 1-5. Approach-Avoidance Gradients for the Total Avoider.

14

PREVALENCE OF DENTAL FEAR

Throughout our lives, few of us are immune from some form of fear or anxiety problem. However, one of the most prevalent fears is of dentistry. Conclusive figures on the prevalence of dental fear are difficult to specify because there have been few studies and they differ in their definition of fear.

In spite of these problems, a review of several survey studies can give us some estimate of the breadth and extent of the problem. For example, one study that sampled the prevalence of various fears in the residents of a moderate sized New England community found that fear of dentists was the fifth most common fear reported (Agras et al., 1969). These investigators found that 19.8 percent of the population reported some moderate degree of fear. In further categorizing fears of a more severe nature, they found that an additional 2.4 percent reported "intense" fear of dentistry, implying that some degree of dental avoidance due to fear was present.

In another large scale study surveying a random sample of the U.S. population, it was found that approximately 6 percent of the respondents reported not receiving needed dental care because of fear (Friedson & Feldman, 1958). Although these two surveys are 15 and 25 years old, more recent surveys seem to bear out the general conclusion that between 4 and 10 percent of the population avoids dentistry due to fear. Kleinknecht and associates recently obtained questionnaire data from some 920 persons concerning their fear and avoidance of dentistry. Although not a random sample, the respondents were from two geographically distinct populations (the states of Florida and Washington) and were of a broad age distribution ranging from 14 to 83 years of age. The questionnaire, called the *Dental Fear Survey*, will be described in detail in Chapter 3. For now, let us look at the responses to three of the questions that pertain to fear and patterns of avoidance. The first question asked was: "Has fear of dentistry ever caused you to put off making an appointment?" Table 1-1 shows the percentages of respondents who indicated each of the five response alternatives. As can be seen in the right-hand column headed "Total," 44.5

TABLE 1-1
Percentages of Respondents Who Report Having Put Off Making a Dental Appointment Due to Fear

Response	Males	Females	Total
	%	%	%
"Never"	60.8	50.6	55.5
"Once or Twice"	19.3	20.6	19.9
"A Few Times"	9.3	12.1	10.7
"Often"	7.7	9.9	9.0
"Nearly Every Time"	2.8	6.3	4.7

$n = 920$

percent of the respondents indicated that they had put off making an appointment at least once due to fear, and 4.7 percent reported doing so "nearly every time" they felt they should make an appointment.

The second question, which addresses a somewhat more severe situation asked: "Has fear ever caused you to cancel or not appear for an appointment that was already made?" Table 1-2 shows that, overall, 14.1 percent reported doing this at least once, and nearly 2 percent reported cancelling either "often" or "nearly every time." These figures, however, may be an underestimate of the actual prevalence of avoidance since the

TABLE 1-2
Percentages of Respondents Who Report Having Cancelled or Not Appeared for a Dental Appointment Due to Fear

Response	Male	Female	Total
	%	%	%
"Never"	90.0	82.3	85.9
"Once or Twice"	7.2	9.5	8.4
"A Few Times"	2.3	4.6	3.6
"Often"	0.5	2.4	1.5
"Nearly Every Time"	0.0	0.8	0.4

$n = 920$

majority of respondents were active patients of dentists who cooperated in this study. A study from Sweden reports that 14 percent of a sample felt dental visits to be "so uncomfortable that they were unable to follow through with treatment" (Seeman & Molin, 1975).

Another question from this survey asked: "All things considered, how fearful are you of having dental work done?" The results of this question, shown in Table 1-3, indicate as stated previously that 74.6 percent reported having at least "a little" fear of dentistry. Further, we can see that 17.5 percent reported their fear to be "much" or "very much." This figure compares closely to that reported by Agras and associates (1969).

In another research study using this same questionnaire, we found that of those patients who indicated their fear to be "much" or "very much" and who subsequently scheduled an appointment, 24 percent failed to appear.

These data clearly indicate dental fear is a widespread occurrence with consequences for patient health and dental practice. Up to 44 percent of persons surveyed report having at some time put off making an appointment due to fear. Moreover, the proportion of cancellations plus "no-shows" resulting from fear is considerable. A sizeable segment of the general population who could benefit from dental care do not receive that care because of fear.

TABLE 1-3
Percentage of Respondents Answering the Question: "All Things Considered, How Fearful Are You of Having Dental Work Done?"

Response	Male	Female	Total
	%	%	%
"Not At All"	29.1	21.8	25.4
"A Little"	40.3	32.7	36.6
"Somewhat"	19.6	21.6	20.5
"Much"	6.1	13.7	10.2
"Very Much"	4.0	10.1	7.3

$n = 920$

PREVALENCE RATES BY AGE AND SEX

The various rates and percentages of persons expressing dental fear shown in the previous section are reflective of the population in general. However, those rates have been shown to differ, depending on other characteristics of the groups. In this section we present information concerning the prevalence of dental fear as it varies according to the person's age and gender.

Age Differences in Fear Prevalence

As is true of most other forms of fears and phobias, as we look at older populations, we find a lower prevalence of fear associated with dentistry.

The data that are available show that the majority of fears begin in the pre-teen years (Kleinknecht et al., 1973; Bernstein & Kleinknecht, 1979; Agras et al., 1969). Fortunately, many of these fears lessen with increasing experience and maturity. Unfortunately, there are persons whose dental fear persists into adulthood. Also adults can develop fear of the dentist.

To provide an overview on the relation between age and the presence and intensity of dental fear, we can look at the figures shown in Table 1-4. This table shows the percentages of 317 persons, grouped into five different age levels, who indicated their degree of dental fear. The scale used here is the one used in Table 1-3.

The left-hand column of Table 1-4 shows a clear trend that as we go from the younger age groups to the older, there is an increasing percentage of respondents who indicate that they have no fear of dentistry. Of the 14 to 21 year old group, 7.7 percent indicate no fear, while 53.7 percent of the group from 50 to 83 report being fearless.

Looking at the far right-hand column, which indicates the percentage who report "very much" fear, we see this trend reversed. Here, 23.1 percent of the youngest age group report "very much" fear while only 3.0 percent of the oldest group indicate this much fear.

If we were to rely only on the overall figures concerning the percentages of persons who report being fearful, we would get a distorted picture.

TABLE 1-4
Percentages of Respondents From Five Age Levels Who Indicated Their Degree of Dental Fear

Age Level	None At All %	A Little %	Some %	Much %	Very Much %	Total %
			Fear Level			
14–21 n = 26	7.7	50.0	11.5	7.7	23.1	100
22–29 n = 104	23.1	32.7	18.3	17.3	8.7	100
30–39 n = 81	34.6	29.6	13.6	11.1	11.1	100
40–49 n = 39	35.9	46.2	10.3	5.1	2.6	100
50–83 n = 67	53.7	29.9	10.4	3.0	3.0	100
Total %	32.8	34.4	13.9	10.4	8.5	100

n = 317

From the sample of patients shown in Table 1-4, the bottom row shows, overall, only 8.5 percent indicating the highest level of fear. This is considerably lower than is true for the youngest group, and much too high for older groups.

In addition to the questionnaire survey data just presented, there are other indictions that older patients, in general, experience less fear than their younger counterparts. This information comes from a study in which patients were evaluated for signs of fear while they were in a dental office and undergoing treatment (Kleinknecht & Bernstein, 1978). In this study, it was found that patients over 40 years of age, compared with those 40 and under, experienced less anxiety during an appointment, reported expecting to experience less pain (prior to treatment), and actually experienced less pain (during treatment) and less physiological arousal as indicated by measures of their sweating response.

Although the data demonstrates that older patients experience less fear than younger patients, keep in mind that these are only general trends and there are many exceptions. We cannot assume that simply because a patient is older, he or she will not be fearful, or that all younger patients will be fearful.

Sex Differences in Fear Prevalence

In dental fear, as with most specific fears and phobias, females generally report being somewhat more fearful than do males. These findings have been borne out in survey questionnaire studies of samples taken from the general population (Agras et al., 1969), college students (Corah et al., 1978; Kleinknecht et al., 1973; Bernstein & Kleinknecht, 1979; Brandon & Kleinknecht, 1982), and dental patients (Kleinknecht & Bernstein, 1978).

The prevalence data previously reported in Tables 1-1, 1-2, and 1-3 show the percentage of males versus females who report varying degrees of dental fear. As can be seen, males predominate in responding to the "not at all" or "never" categories for having put off making an appointment, not appearing for an appointment once made, and general dental fear. Conversely, females are more frequently represented in the response categories indicating greater fear and avoidance.

Similar findings are reported showing females to exhibit more palmar sweating than males when viewing a film of a dental operation (Brandon & Kleinknecht, 1982), and while undergoing dental treatment (Kleinknecht & Bernstein, 1978; Weisenberg et al., 1976).

Although the data reported here consistently find females to demonstrate more dental fear than males, the differences are typically not of such magnitude that one could reliably make individual predictions of which patients are going to be fearful based only on their gender. Nonetheless, there is an overwhelming preponderance of females among patients seeking treatment for dental fear. The percentages of females in such programs range from 75 percent to 86 percent (Bernstein & Kleinknecht, 1978; Klepac et al., 1982; Shaw & Thoresen, 1974). These figures are consistent with our experience at the University of Washington Dental Fear Clinic.* The

* See Appendix A for a brief description of the clinic.

fact that females are more likely than males to seek treatment for their fear should not be too surprising. Women also are the more frequent users of dental services in general.

OBJECTS AND SITUATIONS FEARED

In the preceding section, we discussed dental fear as though it were the whole concept of dentistry that was feared. Although this is the case for some, most people are able to identify specific aspects of dentistry that frighten them most and least. In this section, we describe those situations and procedures that patients report as being most fear arousing. These elements are classified into two general categories: (1) specific situations, instruments, and procedures which are feared, and (2) characteristics of the dental personnel that patients find disturbing.

Instruments and Procedures

Two instruments are consistently cited by patients as producing the most fear or dread: the anesthetic syringe, or "needle," and the "drill." Among virtually all studies conducted that ask patients to rank or rate the elements of dentists most feared, these two instruments come out first and second (Gale, 1972; Kleinknecht et al., 1973; Bernstein et al., 1979). The results of one representative study are shown in Table 1-5. Two hundred students were asked to indicate the amount of fear they experienced when confronted with each of the twelve situations listed. The table shows the average rating (on a 5-point scale) of amount of fear produced by each of these situations, along with the ranking from most (1) to least (5) fearful. Overall, the *feel* of the anesthetic syringe was rated number 1; very close behind was the *sight* of the needle.

The next most fear-provoking aspect of dentistry, ranked number 3, was the sound of the drill, followed by the feeling or vibration from it. The relative ranking of these stimuli holds true whether the respondent reports being highly fearful or not. Although the intensity of fear is greater for the

TABLE 1-5
**Patient Ratings of Fear-Provoking Qualities of
Dental Instruments and Procedures**

	Total		High Fear		Low Fear	
	Mean	*Rank*	*Mean*	*Rank*	*Mean*	*Rank*
Feel the "needle"	3.40	1	4.14	1	2.91	1
See the "needle"	3.31	2	4.08	2.5	2.80	2
Hear the "drill"	3.25	3	4.08	2.5	2.70	3
Feel the "drill"	3.21	4	4.05	4	2.66	4
See the "drill"	2.92	5	3.88	5	2.32	5
Being seated in operatory	2.57	6	3.51	7	1.95	7
Waiting room	2.48	7	3.36	6	1.89	8
Office smell	2.43	8	3.19	9	1.96	6
Seeing dentist	2.39	9	3.30	8	2.78	9
Approaching office	2.20	10	3.10	10	1.60	11
Prophylaxis	1.89	11	2.30	12	1.62	10
Making appointment	1.75	12	2.34	11	1.35	12

Rating Scale: 1 = no fear, 2 = a little, 3 = some, 4 = much, 5 = very much

high fear person, the relative ranking remains the same. This has similarly been found for males and females where females rate each item as causing more fear, but each holds the same relative position.

It has also been shown that the injection produces the most physical fear reaction such as increased heart rate (Hewitt & Stricker, 1977) and increased palmar sweating response (Kleinknecht & Bernstein, 1978; Brandon & Kleinknecht, 1982).

The fear-provoking qualities of the other elements associated with a dental appointment are also of interest. For the most part, the rankings increase the closer one gets to the actual treatment itself. This is an example of the approach-avoidance gradients described earlier. Far from the feared situation, such as making an appointment, the avoidance is less intense than the approach tendency. When approaching the office, smelling the office, sitting in the waiting room and being seated in the operatory, the fear and avoidance increase. If the person's fear becomes too great, the avoidance gradient becomes steeper. They may not follow through with keeping the appointment, which didn't seem so fearful when it was arranged.

The relative rankings of the fear-producing qualities of this sequence of events and specific stimuli holds true whether the person doing the rating is highly fearful or not (Gale, 1972; Kleinknecht, Klepac, & Alexander, 1973; Bernstein & Kleinknecht, 1979). Only the rated intensity of the fear changes. Similarly, males and females tend to rank the situations in the same order, although, as noted earlier, females tend to rate these situations as somewhat more fearful than males.

It should be noted that while these rankings are generally true for most people, there are many important individual exceptions. For example, we have encountered some patients whose fear is primarily of the sensations associated with drilling. But these same patients see the anesthetic syringe as highly positive because they feel it will provide them with anesthesia that will decrease the aversive effects of the drilling. We have seen others who experience virtually no fear to any part of dentistry except that when the anesthetic is about to be injected they become very fearful and defensive. They are quite specifically needle phobic. So, although these general rankings are important for understanding dental fear in general, one cannot assume that each patient has the same problem. Each patient must be evaluated individually for his or her own unique pattern of fears. Chapter 4 will provide the reader with information needed to assess individual patients.

The Dentist

To patients, whether fearful or not, the dentist is clearly the most salient aspect of the dental office. As noted previously, the "needle" and "drill" are the most feared specific stimuli. However, for some patients these may be viewed as extensions of the dentist and influence their perception of the dentist. Hence, for some patients it may be difficult to separate the dentist from the instruments and procedures he or she uses for treatment. Nonetheless, the dentist's professional behavior and personal characteristics are of critical importance in determining patients' views of dentistry.

Information concerning the impact of the dentist on patients comes from a study in which a large number of college students were asked to describe all the factors that contributed to their attitude toward dentistry (Kleinknecht et al., 1979). Far and above all other comments were those that directly referred to the personal and professional behavior of the dentist. Indeed, 91 percent of all respondents made some direct comments relative to the dentist as affecting their attitudes. This focus was present whether the respondent was male or female and whether they reported being fearful or not.

The results showed that among those who considered themselves fearful, 50 percent had negative things to say about the dentist. Among the low fear group, there were 30 percent who had negative comments. The general focus of these negative comments reflected two themes: One centered on personal attributes of the dentist such as "he is impersonal," "nasty," "disinterested," "nervous," "mean," "uncaring," and "cold." The second theme related to what was called "professional behavior" and included comments such as "he is incompetent," "rough," "he yells at me," "would not stop drilling when I told him it hurt," "told me it wouldn't hurt when it really would," "he would strap my arms and legs down." Such comments were succinctly characterized by one of our fearful patients who described his dentist as having the "demeanor of a linebacker and touch of a jackhammer."

It is also of interest to compare patients' reports of pain during treatment relative to comments about the dentist. Although pain is often considered the reason people avoid dentistry, it may not be so clear cut. In the study noted above, one-half of the fearful patients cited the dentist as an important factor in their negative attitudes. Of these, 81 percent did *not* cite pain as affecting their attitudes. For these patients, the dentist himself had greater impact on their fear than pain.

Further supporting the personal impact of the dentist were the comments made by many of the fearless patients that were in stark contrast to the negative statements cited above. Non-fearful, even those who reported having experienced some pain indicated a strong personal liking for their dentist with comments such as: "He is patient, careful, friendly, polite, skilled, professional, warm and caring." We will have more to say concerning these comments about the dentist in Chapter 2 when we discuss the development of dental fear and avoidance.

The Dental Auxiliary

In contrast to the impact of the dentist, the auxiliary personnel were mentioned considerably less often as influencing patients' attitudes toward dentistry. Among the 28 percent who did mention auxiliaries, the vast majority of these comments were of a positive nature. It is of interest that most of the positive comments made were by males who reported themselves as being fearful, whereas the few negative comments were made by female patients. Apparently, the auxiliary personnel are seen by most patients as a positive, soothing and non-threatening aspect of dentistry. Auxiliaries help create atmosphere in the office. Their early contact with the patient may be very important in creating patient comfort.

FEAR OF BEING EMBARRASSED AND BELITTLED

Less commonly, but of significant proportions is the fear some patients express over being embarrassed and belittled by dental personnel. The importance of this fear as a cause of dental avoidance was shown in a study by Gale (1972). Gale found that among 25 situations rated for their fear-producing qualities, the statement: "Dentist tells you that you have bad teeth" was ranked third. In this study, anticipation of such comments was found to be more fear provoking than receiving an injection! Also in this list of 25 situations was the statement: "Dentist laughs as he looks in your mouth," which was ranked as the seventh most fear producing. Although the percentage of cases in which these concerns are found varies from one study to the next, most find that a significant proportion of patients report fear of personal criticism by the dentist (Foresberg, 1966;

Kleinknecht et al., 1973). Such comments by dentists are neither personally nor professionally appropriate and can affect not only the patients' fear and avoidance of dentistry but more generally the public's attitude toward the entire profession.

PATIENT VULNERABILITY AND LOSS OF CONTROL

A final aspect of factors related to patient fear and avoidance is of personal vulnerability and lack of control over the dentist. It is a basic tenet of the psychology that persons under stress experience fear in a potentially threatening situation in which they have little or no control (Davis & Neale, 1981; Miller, 1979; Seligman, 1975). In a stressful situation, the extent to which persons have or, *believe* they have, some personal control over the stressor, there is a corresponding lessening of fear. If pain is involved, the amount of control affects the extent to which pain will be judged as more or less aversive. We believe that this situation has great relevance to patients' reaction to dentistry. Consider, from the patient's point of view, what typically transpires during dental treatment. First, the patient is brought into an operatory, which contains many shining, sharp, and unfamiliar instruments that they vaguely know have the potential to hurt them. He is then reclined in a chair with his head lower than his feet, a very unaccustomed and awkward position, and one that makes it difficult to move the whole body, or to escape. Then, a rubber dam is placed—which prevents him from being able to use speech, the accustomed means of avoiding harm. Further (and possibly more fear provoking), is that with the rubber dam, many patients may have difficulty breathing until they learn they must breathe through their noses. This may be particularly frightening for those who have had no prior experience with a rubber dam and those who have respiratory problems such as asthma. Finally, imagine looking up to see dentist and assistant hovering, holding instruments. In this highly unnatural and restrictive situation, it is not surprising that a person feels vulnerable. The patient is virtually at the mercy of the dentist who is in the position of control and power. Particularly for the apprehensive patient, the perception of the dentist as a powerful professional who is in charge inhibits them from making requests that might increase their comfort. They may feel that it is not their place to question authority.

Given this vulnerability, consider how imposing the instruments and the dentist must appear. It is little wonder that some 75 percent of patients feel at least some fear under these conditions.

Since the dentist must ultimately maintain some control over the situation in order to carry out the treatment, he cannot turn over full control to the patient. In fact, it is not necessary to put the patient in control in order to reduce his or her fear. Numerous studies have shown that the critical element is that the patient *believes* he or she has some control over the potential threat. Therefore, if the dentist can convince the patient through words and actions that he or she can terminate the procedure if it becomes too aversive, less fear and less pain are likely to be experienced. And, the patient's need for exercising any control will also be lessened. This factor of enhancing patients' feeling of control is one of several techniques to be discussed in greater detail in later chapters dealing with treatment and prevention of dental fear.

CONCLUSION

In this first chapter, we have attempted to describe the problem of dental fear, its extent in the general population, and some of the factors from which this fear derives. It was noted that up to three-fourths of the population may experience some fear but that about 10 percent are adversely affected to the extent that they avoid dentistry to the detriment of their oral health.

The sight and sensations of the anesthetic syringe and the drill were shown to be the specific elements most cited as fear provoking. However, the greatest overall impact on patients comes from the personal and professional characteristics of the dentist.

It is also important to remember that there are rational and irrational elements in most cases of dental fear. The reaction is rational to the extent that some pain and discomfort may result. However, we often see reactions that far exceed what would normally be expected under the circumstances of typical dental treatments. When considering these seemingly irrational reactions, it was stated that it is important to view these in their historical contexts. What have the patients' past experiences been with dentistry? How do they currently perceive the dental situation? Even though appearing irrational at the present (such as a panic attack while undergoing a simple prophylaxis), when we learn of the patients' early experiences, their fear may be viewed in a different light.

The current treatment situation may pose little real threat to the patient, but ultimately what determines the reaction will be the patient's *perception* or *belief* concerning what might occur. To the extent that the dentist can understand the patient's perceptions and where they come from, their seemingly irrational behavior will be more understandable. Then the dentist will be in a position to begin changing the patient's negative perceptions and expectations in ways that are more adaptive and health promoting for the patient.

In the process of working to change fearful patients' expectations, it is important that the dentist realize that most fearful patients are, in most other aspects of their lives, rational, normal, and productive individuals. The presence by itself of a seemingly irrational reaction to dentistry should not be taken to imply that the patient is more generally fearful, neurotic, or personally weak.

We believe that it is most productive and accurate to view the fearful dental patient and the problems posed by the fear in the same fashion the dentist views dental disease. That is, the problem is identified and diagnosed, and a rational treatment plan is followed to remedy the problem. All of these therapeutic processes are based on current scientific knowledge. In the chapters that follow, these processes are presented.

QUESTIONS AND EXERCISES

1. Construct and describe an approach-avoidance gradient for a fearful or anxiety-provoking situation in your own life.

2. Consider how you would respond to a new patient who told you that all of his/her prior experiences with dentists were painful and humiliating. What would you say? What would be the main point that you would try to communicate?

3. Describe at least one situation in your life in which you may have very little or no control. How do you feel in each of these situations? Do these situations correspond to how you think dental patients feel?

4. List the major elements that patients report cause them the most anxiety in dentistry. For each item listed, consider what you as a dental professional could do to reduce their fear or apprehension.

TWO

Etiologies of Dental Fear

People are not born fearful. The association of fear with dentistry develops out of socialization and personal learning experiences. Some of these experiences come from direct contact with dentistry while others are communicated indirectly through other people and the mass media.

As noted in Chapter 1, the capacity to experience fear *is* an inborn characteristic. Our nervous systems are "wired" in such a way as to be able to perceive and interpret threatening events and to react physiologically and behaviorally to escape and avoid dangers. However, the attachment of fear to dental stimuli occurs through learning processes that contribute to the development of dental fear. First, each of the processes will be described separately, and then we will present a general model integrating these processes as they typically combine in many cases of dental fear. Finally, we will discuss the implications that this fear development model has for prevention and treatment or "unlearning" of dental fear.

DIRECT EXPERIENCES LEADING TO DENTAL FEAR

The most common means by which patients develop fear and avoidance of dentistry is through direct negative experience in the dental office. These negative experiences may take the form of intense pain or fright and/or may involve negative interpersonal interactions between dentist and patient. In either case, the patient forms an association between dentistry or some aspect of it and unpleasant experiences.

Conditioned Emotional Responses

The following case description of one of our fear patient's reported experiences with dentistry is presented to illustrate how direct experiences can lead to fear and avoidance.

Nora recalled that her early dental experiences were painful and she did not like going at all. However, her parents continued to take her to the dentist on a relatively regular basis. Later, as a 26-year-old adult, Nora experienced an incident that firmly set her into the category of Avoider.

"One day the dentist was filling one of my teeth and accidentally broke off part of another tooth. This really upset me but I knew that I had to go back to get it fixed. At this appointment, the drill slipped from my tooth and drilled a hole in my tongue. I never went back."

Intensely painful and frightening experiences such as this often result in what is called *Conditioned Emotional Responses* (CER). A CER is a conditioned response that has a strong emotional component. It develops when an intensely negative or painful stimulus is applied causing a reflexive emotional response. The negative experience, however, does not occur in isolation. It occurs typically in the presence of some other stimuli with which it becomes associated. The initial stimulus causing pain is called an *Unconditioned Stimulus* (US) because it automatically causes a response, pain or fear. This automatic response is referred to as an *Unconditioned Response* (UR). The UR can elicit an emotional response itself, even without the original painful or frightening stimulation (US). This latter, associated stimulus is called a *Conditioned Stimulus* (CS). The CS then, by itself, acquires the capacity to elicit an emotional response causing the person to experience arousal and avoidance behavior. In the case described above, the dentist, or dentistry in general, became a CS for Nora which caused her to be upset at even the thought of "dentist," and she actively avoided contact with dentistry. We could say that this experience caused her dental avoidance gradient to become higher than her approach gradient. Figure 2-1 shows diagrammatically how a conditioned emotional response can develop.

The CER, developed by associating pain with another stimulus, serves to cause the person to avoid such encounters again. When severe, such reactions are beyond the individual's immediate control. Even though rationally Nora might know that the prospects of being hurt as she

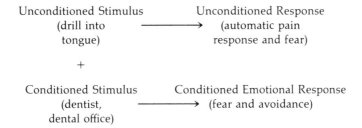

Unconditioned Stimulus   Unconditioned Response
(drill into   ⟶   (automatic pain
tongue)   response and fear)

+

Conditioned Stimulus   Conditioned Emotional Response
(dentist,   ⟶   (fear and avoidance)
dental office)

FIGURE 2-1. A Conditioned Emotional Response to Dentistry.

was the last time are relatively remote, the emotional reaction is still there, automatically. No one, including herself, could talk her out of experiencing the CER.

An additional factor enters at this point, a factor which can actually make the CER stronger, even without re-exposure to the US. As noted above, the person may have a fearful response at the thought of going to the dentist. That is, the CS, thought of a dentist, elicits the emotional response.

When one avoids or escapes from an unpleasant situation, the result is reinforcing: that is, one feels relief. This reinforcement then further serves to keep the individual away from the CS. By not thinking about dentistry, the person avoids the CS and feels less anxiety. Unfortunately, this keeps the person from returning to the dentist where he or she can actually find out that all experiences are not like the one which caused the CER to begin with. As will be discussed later, one of the best ways to eliminate the CER is to gradually re-expose the person to the CS (dental situation) without experiencing the UR (pain). Repeated non-traumatic exposures tend to eliminate the CER.

Dentist Behavior and Patients' Perceptions

In the preceding section, we showed how the conditioning process can elicit reflexive reactions in the patient, based on the association of painful or frightening stimuli, with a person or object that is also present. Such associations are relatively automatic and require no intent. However, as shown in Chapter 1, not all fearful patients report significant painful experiences of this sort, yet they fear and avoid dentistry. Recall that a large percentage felt that the personal and professional characteristics of the dentist were responsible for their fear, independent of pain.

The direct experiences here are of an interpersonal nature. Recall that some fearful patients described their dentists as harsh, uncaring, insulting, or belittling. Interpersonal characteristics are the primary basis on which we form friendships. We prefer to associate with people who are interested in us as persons and who try to make us feel comfortable and at ease. We avoid people who make fun of us, insult us, yell at us, and who hurt us physically or psychologically.

One of our patients described how the behavior of several of his early dentists contributed to his later avoidance. Marvin was self-conscious about his teeth because, as he described them, they were ". . . ugly, irregular and not white."

> I remember one dentist as having bad breath. I only went when it was absolutely necessary. Making an appointment would take me weeks and going would produce a strange dizziness. Being there was worse because the dentist would look at my teeth rather disgustingly and would make nasty remarks. Any pain I ever felt was really of less importance than my fear of being embarrassed and humiliated.

For Marvin, the avoidance and his fear reaction were determined solely on the basis of his dentist's interpersonal behavior toward him. He felt the pain was of little consequence.

The simple rules of interpersonal liking and disliking for others apply even more with dentistry. From the patients' point of view, much more is at stake than just being in the presence of the dentist. As patients, we are captive to the dentist, and many feel that we have little choice in what happens to us once we are in the chair and the rubber dam is placed. Under these conditions, we need to trust the person wielding the potentially harmful instruments. And if that person has not treated us in a manner conducive to liking and trust, we may generalize from his or her personal deficits to question how he or she will treat us physically. "If he

36

treated me badly with his words and manner, how will he treat me physically?" "If he is not concerned with me personally, will he be concerned with how I feel physically?" "If he is clumsy personally, will he be clumsy with his hands?" *Trust* is a major issue for many who fear and avoid dental treatment.

Although such generalization from the interpersonal domain to the professional skill domain may be unwarranted, people do often think in this way. And, if they have no prior experience to go on, their judgment of the dentist will be based on what information is readily available to them—interpersonal behavior. To be more exact, what is most important in this situation is how the patient *perceives* the dentist treating him or her. The accuracy of the patient's perceptions is of little consequence. That is, if the patient perceives the dentist as being demeaning, irrespective of what the dentist actually said or meant, it is the patient's perception that forms the basis for his or her reaction.

In the case of Marvin, for example, we have no way of knowing whether or not his dentist actually made insulting remarks about his teeth and as we will learn in later chapters it does not matter. Marvin may be overly sensitive about his appearance and set to interpret any remark as derogatory, even if it is not meant to be so. The truth of the matter is unknown but the interpretation and its effect are clear.

In summary, the interpersonal behavior of the dentist is one source of fear and avoidance of dentistry. In some cases the fear may be a result of dentists' negative remarks or actions. In others it may be due to patients' tendency to over-generalize or to make faulty interpretations. However, in either situation, the dentist must assume responsibility to ensure that positive communications are made and to take steps to prevent misinterpretation of his or her communication.

INDIRECT EXPERIENCES LEADING TO DENTAL FEAR

Many people are fearful of dentistry even though they have never had direct painful or negative personal experiences themselves. For example, most of our patients come to us afraid of root canal therapy. Although few have previously experienced such treatment they *know* the treatment must be painful and for them this can be a self-fulfilling prophecy. In this section we will discuss two ways in which dental fear can be acquired independently of direct negative dental experiences.

Vicarious and Informational Sources

Much of our learning takes place by observing others and by being instructed in how to perform tasks. We have all seen children imitate their parents and other children, and they are just as likely to imitate bad habits as good. In fact when we want to teach someone something, we say, "Watch me closely so you can do it too!"

We can also become emotionally aroused by observing others experience an emotion. Being around someone who is extremely happy or joyous gives us a good feeling. Seeing someone extremely sad or witnessing a tragic event makes us feel similarly sad. Who has not been frightened by a horror movie, even though it is an actor on the screen who is being pursued by the monster? We are not being chased, but we have come to *vicariously* identify with the hero or heroine and think of their experiences as though they were our own. Such sympathetic or vicarious emotional arousal happens particularly strongly if we know or like the person we are observing.

Dental fear can be similarly communicated. Probably the most common source of this vicarious fear development is from parents to children. Research (see Chapter 10) has shown that many fearful children have fearful parents as well. Through hearing parents talk of their fear or dislike of dentistry and/or through seeing their parents react adversely to dentistry, children can acquire both the information that says "dentists are to be avoided" *and* they can acquire the parents' emotional reaction to the whole concept of dentistry.

From our experience, many parents are fully aware of this vicarious process. Many of our fear patients seek treatment for their fear so that they will not pass it on to their children. Recall the example of Joan given in Chapter 1. Her dental fear began by observing her mother being upset and crying at the dentist's office—before she herself had ever gone. Years later when she came for treatment, her expressed reason was that she wanted to overcome her fear so she would not transmit it to her two children, as her mother had to her.

The Mass Media

Another vehicle by which specific fear information is communicated is through the many forms of mass media. Cartoons seen in newspapers and magazines are full of characterizations of dentists as inflicters of torture. The cartoon shown below is one example. Just as individuals can communicate information, so can such pictures. The message of this cartoon is

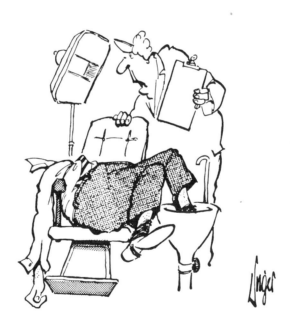

"Dr. Burns says you need two more appointments."

clearly spelled out: "If you go to the dentist, you can expect to be hurt." Such information, or "misinformation," can serve to reinforce any other similar messages one may have received from parents or others. Consider the potential effect of these two sources of fear information together. Before directly experiencing dentistry personally, the reader of this media will have an expectation that, if and when they do go, traumatic things will occur. With this expectation, he or she will enter with considerable anticipatory anxiety. Then, even mildly uncomfortable stimulations may be perceived as painful so their worst fears are in fact realized. Dentistry will be painful. (This relationship between being aroused and the enhanced perception of pain will be described in greater detail in Chapter 3.)

Stimulus Generalization

We introduced stimulus generalization earlier in this chapter. It is the process by which a person conditioned to respond to one stimulus (CS) associated with pain or trauma will also respond emotionally to similar stimuli or situations. Through this process, some people, who have never had direct negative experiences with dentistry, might respond adversely to elements of the dental situation that are reminiscent of another similar situation in which they have been traumatized. One common situation to which this applies is medical/surgical procedures. Such responses are often very perplexing to the dental personnel and even to patients. To them it does not seem rational that just because one situation was aversive, another should be as well.

An excellent example of one such case of generalization was described by Borland (1962).

> Many years ago I did some extensive dental procedures in the mouth of a young housewife who fainted every time we began a session in the chair. This continued for a number of appointments until one day I returned a few minutes late from a luncheon club meeting to find the patient already in the chair. I went into the operating room in a business suit and injected the

40

anesthetic, and waited for her to faint. She did not, but on the next appointment, when I was dressed in a white jacket, she fainted as reliably as ever. Subsequently, I always wore a sport shirt rather than a white jacket when treating this patient, and the fainting stopped. Discussions with the patient after the treatment was completed revealed that she had been terribly frightened when she had undergone a tonsillectomy as a child, and that she still had occasional nightmares about this in which the element that she described the most vividly and with the most feeling was the white uniforms worn by the doctors and nurses. This patient was not reacting to *me*, but to a very distorted *percept* of me—a percept whose distortion seemed to be particularly mediated by the white uniforms. When this element was removed from the situation, her perception of the situation was determined more by its real characteristics and less by the attributes of an old experience of which it reminded her. Her feelings, from which she defended herself by fainting, were quite appropriate for the original situation but quite inappropriate for the contemporary one. (p. 188)

This account of stimulus generalization illustrates several points important to a full understanding of etiology and treatment for dental fear. First, it shows that one does *not* have to have been harmed by or in the presence of a dentist to react adversely to dentistry. This reaction itself was in no way the fault of a dentist. Secondly, it shows that individuals may have very different reactions to fear. In this case, rather than showing the more common symptoms associated with arousal of the sympathetic branch of the ANS such as increased heart rate, respiration and the like, she appeared to show arousal of the parasympathetic branch, resulting in a drop in heart rate and blood pressure and syncope. Although less common among fear reactions than sympathetic response, this parasympathetic arousal is often seen among those with fears of blood and injury (Connolly, Hallan, & Marks, 1975). A third point is Borland's interpretation of her responding to a "distorted percept." Rather than characterizing her reaction as *distorted*, it is more accurate to think of this in terms of her reacting to a specific stimulus of white coat, which was highly similar to the situation in which she acquired this CER. We need not imply that the patient's perceptions were in any way deviant; knowing her medical history, the reaction is realistic. Had a full medical history been taken earlier in which the patient could recount her experience, the dentist could have prevented her syncope from the outset.

It is partially for reasons of stimulus generalization that many dentists have changed the atmosphere of their offices. Rather than sterile-looking white offices and uniforms, today we see more soft comfortable interior decorating with carpeting, colored chairs, art work, and plants. The dentist and auxiliaries are often found to wear colorful, patterned attire. Few stimuli remain that are clearly associated with the traditional dental and medical settings. We have had many fearful patients who have avoided dentistry for years comment on how these changes made them feel less threatened and more comfortable. However, these new surroundings cannot *prevent* the development of fear. Should a patient be exposed to painful or fear-eliciting stimuli in this setting, it could become a CS for fear as well.

Another common source of fear reactions to dentistry caused by stimulus generalization is an experience that virtually all children go through receiving immunization injections. This may be one of the reasons that fear of the local anesthetic injection is so prominent as shown in Chapter 1. The following example illustrates this process of fear developing in one situation and generalizing to another.

Joe was a 20-year-old college student when he was referred for fear treatment to one of us by a general practice dentist. Joe had avoided dentists for at least 10 years. When he developed a severe toothache, he got up his courage, made an appointment and went to the referring dentist. However, when the dentist attempted the anesthetic injection, Joe jerked his arms up in front of his face and pulled his legs up to his chest. He curled up into a ball. He wasn't going to allow the injection. The dentist then administered nitrous oxide and Joe appeared much more relaxed and reported that he was ready. As the syringe approached his mouth, his reaction was the same. He curled up again and would not allow the injection.

When interviewing Joe prior to treating him for the fear, he described where this reaction originated. As a child about age 10, he recalled standing in line at school where all the children were receiving immunizations. When he got near the front of the line, he observed the child ahead of him being injected. The child screamed and jerked, and the syringe separated from the needle, which stayed in his arm. Joe vividly recalled seeing the child crying with the needle dangling from his arm. Joe ran away and would not allow the nurse to give him his injection. As a result, he avoided dentistry altogether. As a teenager when his mother made dental appointments for him, he conveniently "forgot" them and never went. Not only did he avoid going to the dentist, he avoided even *thinking* about going.

Joe's fear was acquired vicariously through observation and even though he was not hurt by the injection, the fear developed and generalized to all situations involving needles, including dentistry.

These two examples illustrate how fears, developed in medical settings, generalize to dentistry. Although the dentist in both cases could do nothing about the origins of these reactions, by appropriate assessment methods initiated prior to treatment, the dentist could have identified the source and thus would have been in a better position to deal with the fear reaction at an earlier stage of treatment. Techniques for assessing such problems and for treating them will be described in the subsequent chapters.

Helplessness and Lack of Control

The last two sources contributing to dental fear are extremely important, though somewhat less specific than those discussed thus far. Both involve more thinking and interpretaton of situations by the patient. The first to be discussed involves situations in which the individual experiences a sense of helplessness over something that may cause them discomfort, pain, or injury.

Patients' feelings of helplessness and vulnerability were mentioned in Chapter 1 as one of the situations that patients feared and was related to reasons for avoidance. Here we will expand on this very important topic because we feel it touches the heart of dental fear. Feelings of helplessness are important in their own right as a cause of fear and are intimately involved in affecting one's reactions to the previously described sources of fear. Moreover, elimination of these feelings is critical to overcoming fear. Before proceeding with our discussion of lack of control, it is important to indicate what is meant by *control*. A simple, but useful, definition is given by Thompson (1981) who states that control is ". . . the belief that one has at one's disposal a response that can influence the aversiveness of an event" (p. 89).

A critical element of this definition and the discussion to follow is the word *belief*. If the person believes he or she has no means of influencing the negative effect, then there will be the perception of helplessness and lack of control. Extensive research has shown that such feelings lead to fear. The opposite belief, that one *does* have control, can lead to lessened fear. This is the case whether or not the person in fact has control. It is effective so long as they believe they have control. This effect was clearly demonstrated in a study by Geer and his colleagues (1970), in which a group of subjects initially were given a series of 10 painful electric shocks. Throughout the experiment, subjects' electrodermal responses were measured as a physiological indicator of their anticipatory anxiety prior to each shock. They were also required to press a button immediately following each shock. They were told initially that this would be a measure of their reaction time.

After the first 10 shocks were given, half of the subjects were told that if they pressed the button quickly enough they could shorten the duration of the shock from 6 to 3 seconds. Actually, unknown to the subjects, the experimenters arranged all shocks to be 3 seconds, but this statement created the belief that it was the subjects themselves who controlled the duration. The other half of the subjects were simply told that the remaining 10 shocks would be shorter.

During the second series of 10 shocks, the group who were led to believe that their speed of responding was responsible for the shorter shocks—that is, who felt they controlled the duration—showed dramatically less physical arousal to the shocks than those who did not believe they had control. In this study, both groups received exactly the same number and duration of shocks. The only differences responsible for one group showing less anxiety was their belief (erroneous) that they could do something to influence the shock.

The foregoing study demonstrated one means by which control might be exerted over an aversive event. There are other forms of control that also have direct relevance of dental fear and anxiety. These four types of control that were described by Thompson (1981) are: Behavioral, Cognitive, Informational, and Retrospective.

BEHAVIORAL CONTROL. This category includes those situations in which the person believes he or she can make some behavioral response that will terminate, shorten, or lessen an aversive event. The study cited above was an example of behavioral control because the subjects believed that a rapid button press would shorten the duration of the shock. Those who were not told they had such a response available believed they had no control and showed more fear arousal. An example often used by dentists is to tell the patient they can signal him by raising their finger or hand to indicate that a procedure is becoming stressful. Again, we must emphasize that all that is necessary for this control to reduce anxieties is for patients to *believe* they can control the aversiveness of the event.

The feelings of lack of behavioral control are often cited by our fear patients as either being the cause of or contributing to their dental fear. They report that "... the dentist wouldn't stop when it hurt." "He wouldn't give me more Novacaine when I asked." Such incidents would easily lead patients to believe that they have no control. In fact, the only control they believe they have is not to go to the dentist.

COGNITIVE CONTROL. Cognitive control involves something that patients can do mentally that will lessen the aversiveness of the stimulation or their reaction to the stimulation. Here we will focus on the *lack* of cognitive control or the inability of patients to control negative thoughts concerning what might happen to them while undergoing dental treatment. Fearful patients often report that both prior to and during dental treatment, they experience repeated negative or "catastrophizing" thoughts that serve to keep them anxious.

In a recent study, an attempt was made to identify what fearful and

45

non-fearful persons thought about and said to themselves while viewing a videotaped simulation of a dental restoration. Persons who characterized themselves, prior to the study, as fearful, reported thinking "catastrophizing" thoughts. That is, they thought of all the possible negative or catastrophic things that could happen such as, "What if the needle slips," "This is going to hurt," "When will he stop," etc. Of the subjects in this study who experienced catastrophizing thoughts, 87 percent were from the high dental fear group. In contrast, the vast majority of those in the low fear group reported either no specific thoughts or used coping thoughts that helped them control any anxiety such as: "I can trust this dentist," "It's really not that bad, it could be worse." Others recalled pleasant memories, some from dentists, others from being in comfortable places. These coping thoughts provided the subjects with some cognitive control over a potentially negative situation. In contrast, catastrophizing subjects who felt they had no control, based on their thought reactions, continued to be fearful and reported that the film made them much more anxious and caused them more physiological arousal than was experienced by those who used some cognitive control strategy.

INFORMATION. The information that gives the person under stress some feeling of control includes what the situation or procedure is like, warnings that the aversive event is about to occur, and what sensations the person is likely to experience. This issue boils down to how much to tell the patient about what will transpire during treatment.

The extent to which such information or lack of it affects one's reaction to specific stimuli depends on several complex factors. We will start by discussing the simplest case: that of providing a warning or signal that something is about to occur. Seligman (1975) contends that it is important to know when an aversive event is going to happen. When it is clear to persons that they will be signaled whenever something negative will happen, this amounts to a "danger signal." On the other hand, if it is clear that all danger will be signaled, absence of the danger signal or warning can be taken as a "safety signal." Therefore, when the safety signal is present there is no need to be anxious. Therefore, the anxiety or fear arousal will only be periodic and short lasting. Being in a potentially threatening situation and never knowing when the actual negative event will occur keeps one in a continuous state of anticipatory anxiety. Lack of any information results in the patient being uncertain about what might occur. Another way of viewing this is a fear of the unknown. That is, the person is anxious because he does not know what the safety signals are.

We have seen some patients who report that their dislike (fear) of dentists stems from the fact that the dentist never told them when he would give them the local anesthetic injection. "My dentist would tell me to look the other way. Then when I looked back, he had the needle ready to stick me. He was really sneaky and I didn't like that."

Under such conditions of uncertainty, the patient knew she would receive an injection but was never sure just when. This kept her in a constant anxiety state that contributed to her overall fear of dentistry. Distrust develops in such situations.

Another aspect involving information given to patients involves providing them with detailed accurate information concerning what procedures are to occur and what sensations they are likely to experience from the procedures. Presumably, if one does not know what is going to happen and what to expect, there will not only be prior, anticipatory anxiety with the patient wondering or "catastrophizing" about which might occur, there will also be the startle or surprise when it does occur. If the patient is prepared for what is to come, fear of the unknown will be lessened and the patient will need to rely less on his or her imagination to determine what will happen. Also, once experiencing an anticipated sensation, he or she will know that the experience is normal, rather than something to be concerned about.

The research concerning whether or not to provide patients with information generally shows that lack of information may result in fear. However, a couple of other factors qualify this conclusion. First, the positive effects of information tend to be enhanced when the patient is not only given the information, but is also given a way of coping with any response that might result from this information (Thompson, 1981). In Chapter 6, we discuss how information and a breathing exercise were helpful for a patient who had refused anesthetic injections her entire adult life.

A second qualification of the effects of information on anxiety is that *some* people prefer *not* to know *what* will happen or *when*. Giving these people too much information may actually make them more fearful. Consequently, it may be useful to ask patients how much information they would like to have. Probably the majority of patients prefer to be informed, and for them, the information appears to reduce fear. Not informing them will make them fearful as it did this patient: "I am afraid of pain and the unknown. Before childbirth and before I had surgery, my doctor explained everything that was going to happen and I wasn't afraid anymore. No dentist has ever explained anything to me and I'm afraid 'cause I don't know what will happen."

RETROSPECTIVE CONTROL. This final category of control may not be control in the sense that we usually use the term. Rather, it refers to the patient identifying the cause of an aversive event, after it has occurred. Once a patient can attribute the cause to something rational it gives the event more meaning and can reduce the long-term reactions to it. For example, an avoider who has been treated for his fear may become aware that anticipation, not the dental treatment itself, is his biggest problem. At this point, he is well on his way to being able to control future anticipation. For another variation on retrospective control, consider a patient who is required to undergo extensive restoration treatment that may be quite uncomfortable, painful, and anxiety provoking. If such patients identify the reason they are in this condition as their previous neglect of their oral health care, they know the responsibility lies with themselves, not the dentist nor the instruments. Further, knowing that we are personally to blame tells us what we must do in the future to prevent its recurrence. In this sense, through retrospect, the situation has meaning and order and provides a sense of control in that we know what to do to avoid or lessen future discomfort.

The Meaning of the Event

The foregoing discussion of the effects of lack of control indicate that when most people are about to experience an unpleasant event and when they believe they have no means of influencing the event, the result is fear and greater pain. A useful unifying concept to tie together the several methods of control is to consider the *meaning* that the event has for the person. If the meaning of the impending event is: "I will experience more discomfort (fear, pain, embarrassment) than I am capable of tolerating *and* I have no means of escape or control," the result is fear. Conversely, *if in the face of threat, he or she can exercise control if desired, the meaning of the situation changes to one of tolerability with less fear.*

Using this perspective, we can analyze the development of dental fear in terms of what dentistry means to patients. To begin this analysis, consider the question: "Where does the meaning come from?" In brief, meaning develops out of our direct and indirect experiences with dentists and similar situations: through Conditioned Emotional Responses, dentists' personal and professional characteristics, from information communicated by friends, family, and the media. Through these experiences dentistry takes on meaning as either something positive and approachable or something negative that is to be avoided. As part of the process, we develop our beliefs about our ability to control the situation, if necessary.

If our experiences have been painful or frightening *and* we believe we have no control, dentistry will be something to fear and to avoid. On the other hand, if our experiences have been positive and/or if we feel we can effectively control any aversiveness, then we can approach it with little or no fear. For the patient whose experiences have been positive and who believes he or she is in the hands of a highly skilled and competent dentist, the issue of control becomes moot. In fact some patients report that when they are under the care of a professional who is perceived as attempting to minimize harm to the patient, personal control is not even preferred (Thompson, 1981). This patient says, "Do whatever is necessary—you're the doctor."

The preceding analysis then brings us back to a central issue mentioned previously: that the dentist is the most salient feature of dentistry, and it is from the dentist's behavior that much of the meaning of dentistry is derived. With this background concerning the causes of dental fear and the importance of control over aversive situations, let us now analyze the dental experiences of Harry, who prior to coming to our fear treatment program had avoided dentistry for eight years.

> My first recollection is having teeth pulled. I was around age 6. I was taken to the hospital and had some permanent teeth cut out or pulled out. I can still remember the mask coming down over my face and the strong smell of ether. Then I had a technicolor dream of a train running over me which I can still remember. I remember waking and everyone being nice but being scared.
>
> Later when I was 7 or 8, the dentist didn't give me enough Novocaine when filling my teeth and I cried out. He slapped his hand over my mouth hard and said "shut up."
>
> Then about 8 years ago, I had a terrible toothache and I went to another dentist. He proceeded to pull the tooth under Novocaine but the pain was excruciating. So he stopped with the tooth half out and cracked and told me to go to an oral surgeon. I can still remember the pain while waiting to have that tooth cut out.

Several points from Harry's history with dentistry illustrate the concepts discussed earlier. Harry's first experience with dentistry at age six was very frightening. He had no control over what was happening, and even though he did not recall any specific pain, his perception of what happened was that he had teeth *cut* out—a frightening thought to a young child. Although the people were "being nice," he was still scared. Dentistry now had some meaning to him.

His next experience involved pain at the hands of the dentist. Not only did he have no control, he believed that he was abused by the dentist for attempting to control the situation. The meaning of dentistry was clearer to him by then.

Finally, his last appointment involved severe pain and no opportunity to control it. The pain was extended by his having to wait for the oral surgeon to complete the extraction. Harry had all of the conditions for the development of dental fear: fear of the unknown, extensive and extended pain, perceived abuse and unprofessional behavior by the dentist, *and* no means by which he could control either his or the dentist's reactions or behavior. By this time, dentistry had a very clear meaning to Harry.

A MODEL OF DENTAL FEAR ACQUISITION

In the preceding sections we described the various processes that contribute to a patient's fear development. In this section we integrate these processes into a comprehensive model. This model will serve as a basis for guiding our discussion throughout this text and points to methods for the prevention and treatment of dental fear. As can be seen in the schematic presentation of the Model in Table 2-1, the two major factors involved in fear development are: (1) the patients' prior experiences with dentistry, direct and indirect, and (2) the patients' perceptions of whether or not they have or could have, if desired, control over what will happen to them. Each of the four combinations will be discussed in turn.

TABLE 2-1
A Model of Dental Fear

Dental Experiences	Patient Perceived Control	
	Yes	No
Positive	—no fear	—no fear
	—approach	—approach
	—highly positive attitudes	—highly positive attitudes
Negative	—some anticipatory anxiety possible	—fear
	—no or little fear	—avoidance
	—mostly approach	—highly negative attitude
	—attitude highly positive to mildly negative	

Positive Experiences and Perceived Control

As suggested in the previous sections, patients whose experiences with dentistry have been positive and who have been led to believe they can control any negative or painful stimulation are unlikely to experience dental fear. They will not avoid dentistry, and their general attitudes toward dentists and dentistry as a profession will be highly positive. Factors contributing to this positive outlook on dentistry would likely involve early encouragement and positive communication by parents and actual dental experiences of a positive, relatively unpainful nature by a dentist and staff who communicate to the patient that he or she is seen as an individual and will be treated with respect and will have, if desired, some say in their treatment. The result would be a satisfied patient who is unlikely to miss appointments *and* a patient who is cooperative and a pleasure to treat.

Positive Experiences and No Perceived Control

Patients falling into this category of experiences may be very similar to their counterparts with positive experiences and control. They are not likely to experience fear so they probably will not avoid dentists in the future. Given their experiences of a positive nature, which would likely contribute to their liking and trusting their dentists, the issue of control becomes less relevant. Recall in our previous discussion of research on perceived control that some people who believe they are in the care of a competent and trustworthy practitioner may actually prefer to relinquish control. In either case, whether or not they actually prefer to leave control in the hands of the provider, the fact that they have little or no need to control the situation renders the control issue moot.

Negative Experiences and Perceived Control

Those patients who have had some of the negative experiences noted previously but who do believe they have control present a more mixed picture. Here we need to describe several alternatives encompassed in these conditions. For many in this group, there is likely to be at least some level of anxiety. The extent of the anxiety would largely be determined by the number and intensity of their past experiences. If a patient has had several negative experiences at the hands of a dentist other than the one who currently provides the sense of control, the patient would likely experience some anxiety. This might last until he or she was able to actually experience some measure of control. In fact we have found that approximately one-fourth of low fear patients who describe early painful experiences have changed to dentists with whom they feel more comfortable (Bernstein, Kleinknecht, & Alexander, 1979).

Another situation that falls into this category involves those patients who have had to undergo extensive restoration and describe the experience as very painful, but do not develop fear as a result. The surveys noted above indicated that some non-fearful patients described early painful dental experiences. Approximately 40 percent of these patients also made complimentary comments about their dentists. Our interpretation of this is that it is not necessarily pain experiences themselves that cause fear. Rather, in the presence of pain, the factor that determines whether or not fear will result is the manner in which the dentist deals with the patient's pain. As one low fear patient from our survey described her experiences, "Dr. Rosen was great. Whenever it would hurt real bad, he would stop until I felt better before starting again." Pain experienced by a patient in control is not likely to lead to fear. It is the interaction of the dentist and the patient which determines whether fear will result from pain.

Negative Experiences and No Perceived Control

With these two conditions present, we feel that fear is the automatic outcome. The patient who has been led to believe that dentistry is painful, whose actual experience is traumatic, and who has no feeling of control over the situation will develop fear, avoid dentistry, and have negative attitudes toward the professon. From the dentist's point of view, when and if such patients appear, they will be difficult to treat and stressful for the dental personnel. However, it is primarily the treatment of this group for which this book is written. It is our belief and experience, supported by research, that the fear can be treated and that such persons can be introduced into the ranks of satisfied, cooperative, and enjoyable patients.

A MODEL OF DENTAL FEAR TREATMENT

To complement the preceding model of dental fear development, we now introduce a model of dental fear treatment. This model is essentially the converse of the fear development model presented above and will serve as the guiding basis for the several treatment approaches to be described in detail in Chapters 5–9.

The model derives from a cognitive, social learning approach to fear reduction, as described by Albert Bandura (1977). It is cognitive in that we believe that an important element in determining dental fear behavior and its change is how the person *thinks* about themselves in the feared situation. It involves social learning in that new ways of thinking and behaving (e.g., fearlessness) are learned. And this learning takes place in a social context involving information acquired from others, especially dental personnel. Dentistry, as noted in the previous section, is as much of a social situation involving interaction with others as it is a technical process.

In its basic form, this model proposes that fear and avoidance behavior are acquired through a variety of direct and indirect experiences as described earlier. These experiences and their resultant perceptions of dentistry provide the patient with certain *expectations* about what will occur. If the expectation is that "I will experience pain, humiliation, and/or be unable to control myself or the situation, "anxiety, fear, and avoidance will result. In other words, if a patient's past experience has led him to believe that what he will encounter at the dental office is beyond his ability to cope, he will experience fear.

Given this conceptualization of fear development, the focus of treatment is to change patients' expectations about what they will experience and their ability to cope with what they do experience.

The model also proposes a variety of means by which these expectations can be changed to enable the person to enter or re-enter dentistry and to feel confident of his ability to cope. Here, we will briefly outline the

TABLE 2-2
Outline of the Treatment Model:
Sources of Expectancy Change and Fear Reduction

Direct Experiences

1. Exposure to non-traumatic dental treatment
2. Patient experiences sense of control if desired

Indirect Experiences

1. Observation of others undergoing non-traumatic dental experiences (live or on video)
2. Receiving information on modern dental treatment

Development of Coping Skills

1. Learning to relax in dental treatment
2. Learning to pace and deep breathing
3. Learning positive self-statements
4. Avoiding negative "catastrophizing" statements
5. Learning to distract self
6. Learning to talk to dental personnel to exercise control if needed

---

types of experiences that can contribute to changes in their beliefs or expectations. Paralleling our fear development model, we can separate these into direct and indirect experiences. A third category of experience is added: learning coping skills. As we will see, these several types of experiences often need to be combined in order to most effectively change one's expectations and fear. An outline of this fear treatment model is shown in Table 2-2.

Sources of Expectancy Change

DIRECT EXPERIENCES. The most reliable and most powerful means of reducing fear and changing one's expectancy about dentistry is direct positive experiences. In the same way that direct negative experiences create fear and negative expectations, direct positive experiences show the patient that what he will experience will be counter to his expectations of trauma. This actual exposure to dentistry without negative consequences serves to alter his future expectancy of trauma and thus beings to extinguish conditioned emotional reactions.

As with any other learning process, complete change may take several exposures to be fully effective. Further, since fearful patients will hold negative expectations, they may initially feel unable to cope with a full treatment appointment. Consequently, the dental personnel may need to structure initial appointments of short duration and minimal treatment. As patients experience success in coping with each stage, the expectancy of their ability to handle later ones increases, and fear decreases. Chapter 5 contains a discussion of planning dental treatment to provide short positive experiences.

INDIRECT EXPERIENCES. Indirect experiences which communicate to the patient that negative expectancies are exaggerated can also contribute to fear reduction. Vicarious experiences, such as observing others undergoing non-traumatic and positive dental treatment, can serve this purpose. Such modeling procedures have been widely and successfully used, especially with children (Melamed et al., 1975; Williams et al., 1983). Other indirect exposures that serve to change expectancies include reading about "modern dentistry," seeing film strips describing what actually occurs, and simply talking to others who have had positive experiences with trustworthy dentists. Although these latter procedures are unlikely by themselves to eliminate fear entirely, they may provide sufficient change in expectancy to allow the fearful patient to take the first step toward direct exposure.

LEARNING COPING SKILLS. The final category of treatment procedures to change fear is aimed directly at enhancing the patients' perception of their own abilities to cope with dentistry. Included here are techniques for learning relaxation skills to be applied before and during treatment; training in making coping and positive self-statements to replace negative catastrophizing statements; distraction procedures; and training in talking to dental personnel to facilitate feelings of personal control over what is happening to them. These skills are discussed in Chapters 6-9.

In general, this model proposes a variety of procedures aimed at changing the patients' perceptions of and experiences with dentistry. In most cases, several of these procedures may need to be combined for successful fear treatment. The indirect experiences and training in coping skills may be necessary to bring the patient to the point where he or she is ready to directly experience non-traumatic dentistry. We believe that it is through this direct exposure to dentistry, conducted by observant, trustworthy, and concerned dental personnel, that significant expectancy and hence fear change occurs.

CONCLUSION

In this chapter we have outlined the major processes by which patients develop their fear and avoidance of dentistry. It was shown that direct experiences with painful or frightening dental situations could lead to *conditioned emotional responses* in which the dentist or some aspect of dentistry became associated with the trauma. Through these experiences, elements of the dental situation acquired the capacity to automatically elicit an emotional response, even without the original unconditioned stimulus being experienced.

Another source of direct experience leading to fear concerned the *dentists' behavior* toward the patient. Such dentist behaviors as belittlement, scolding, or an impersonal, uncaring attitude also contribute to patients' fear and lack of trust. Further it was noted that the critical element here was not just how the dentist behaved, but how the patient *perceived* or interpreted what the dentist did or said.

Some people appear to be fearful of dentistry even though they themselves have had no direct negative experiences. For these, we discussed several types of indirect experiences that contribute to fear. These included *vicarious experiences* and *information* communicated by others, which led patients to believe that dentistry could harm them. Similarly, it was noted that the *mass media* with jokes and cartoons depicting the horrors of dentistry were abundant.

Other patients who have never directly experienced dental trauma may have acquired their fear of dentistry through *stimulus generalization*.

Such patients may have experienced fear and/or pain in other medical settings and because of the similarity with dentistry, the original reaction can be elicited by the dental situation.

Important in its own right and contributing to the other sources of dental fear are the feelings of *helplessness* and *perceived lack of control* over potentially threatening situations. Four types of patient control were mentioned and the effects of their absence were described: *behavioral control, cognitive control, informational control,* and *retrospective control.* The sense of control that a patient felt or did not feel contributed to the *meaning* that the situation or event had for the patient. If the dental situation meant to the patient that he or she would experience discomfort and have no means to control or escape it, the result would be heightened anxiety or fear.

A *model of dental fear acquisition* was described that combined patients' experiences with the notions of perceived control. It was noted that when negative experiences were present *and* the patient felt no sense of control, fear was the likely outcome.

Finally, a model of dental fear treatment was presented that focused on changing patients' *expectations* concerning what might occur at a dental office. It was noted that these expectations of trauma were most effectively countered by gradually providing patients with direct positive dental experiences in which they are given a sense of control, both over the procedures being conducted and over their own reactions to those procedures.

QUESTIONS AND EXERCISES

1. Recall either the first time you went to the dentist or the earliest appointment that you can remember. How did you feel? What were the reasons for your feelings? What do you recall about the dentist? the auxiliaries? the instruments? the office? What were the positive aspects of this experience? What were the negative aspects? What would you have done differently if you had been the dental professional in that situation?

2. Recall the last time you had any medical or dental treatment. What were the salient features of that appointment? What things did you like and what did you dislike about the facility or provider?

3. From your own experiences with dental patients or with friends who have expressed being fearful of dentistry, how closely do their accounts or stories mesh with those described in this chapter? Were they basically the same or were there other causes?

4. What is the difference between being at a horror movie in which you experience vicarious fear and a situation such as observing someone about to be actually injured? One dimension of difference is that you know one is real and one is not. What other similarities and differences are there in these two situations?

5. Considering the model of treatment described at the end of Chapter 2, outline the elements of a treatment plan for treating someone who is fearful of swimming, or fearful of heights.

6. Recall how you felt the first time you saw a patient as a dental professional. How did it feel? What thoughts were in your mind? Were you anxious or fearful? If so, why? Do you think that patients feel similarly when they come to you for the first time?

7. Recall a situation in which you felt embarrassed or put down. How did this occur? Why did this situation embarrass you? How did it affect you the next time you were in the same or similar situation? What could or should have been done differently by you or by the other person involved? How might similar situations occur with dental patients?

8. Ask ten persons whether or not they have ever been fearful or apprehensive of dentistry. Among those who say they have, ask what the causes were of their fear. Were they direct experiences or indirect experiences? Of those who were once fearful but are not currently, what was responsible for their getting over their fear?

THREE

Pain and Pain Control for Fearful Patients

As we discussed in Chapter 2, unpleasant direct and indirect experiences play a major role in the etiology of dental fear. Moreover, pain control is an important clinical requirement in the treatment of such patients. Thus, in large part this chapter is intended as a bridge between our discussion of the problem of fear and its treatment.

There are, however, two additional reasons for a special chapter de-

HERMAN®

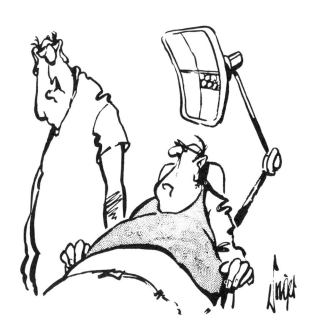

"Why don't you have a good scream and get it over with."

voted to this subject and placed at this point in the text. First, although pain control is not a new subject for the dentist, we have found that many inaccuracies and errors occur in this area, suggesting that dentists are failing to adopt new information. Second, many dental personnel see anxiety control, especially the modalities of nitrous oxide, oral premedication, and IV sedation, as the *primary* means of treating the fearful patient. We hope to describe what we have found to be the appropriate uses of these drugs while also strongly suggesting complementary behavioral strategies.

CONCEPTUALIZING PAIN

This chapter includes a definition and theories of pain and its relationships to fear and anxiety, cultural factors related to pain, coping strategies, and personality factors. We also discuss local anesthestics and other drugs used in dentistry such as nitrous oxide and diazepam. The first section of this chapter defines what we mean by pain, specifies two theories of pain and their clinical implications, and establishes the relationship between anxiety and pain. If pain is not just a sensation, what is it? That question cannot be answered simply because pain is a complex phenomenon. Sternbach (1968) described pain as an abstract concept that refers to (1) a personal, private sensation of hurt; (2) a harmful stimulus that signals current or impending tissue damage; and (3) a pattern of responses that operates to protect the organism from harm. In some respects, pain is a sensation and in other respects it is a psychological phenomenon that allows us to escape or avoid trauma.

Consider the definition of pain arrived at by an international group of experts and published by *Pain* in 1979.

> ... An unpleasant sensory and emotional experience associated with actual or potential tissue damage, or described in terms of damage.
> ... Pain is always subjective. Each individual learns the application of the word with experiences related to injury in early life. Biologists recognize that those stimuli which cause

pain are liable to damage tissue. Accordingly, pain is that experience which we associate with actual or potential tissue damage. It is unquestionably a sensation in a part or parts of the body but is also always unpleasant and therefore also an emotional experience. Experiences which resemble pain, e.g., pricking, but are not unpleasant, should not be called pain. . . .

Many people report pain in the absence of tissue damage or any likely pathophysiological cause; usually this happens for psychological reasons. There is no way to distinguish their experience from that due to tissue damage if we take the subjective report. *If they regard their experience as pain and if they report it in the same ways as pain caused by tissue damage, it should be accepted as pain.* (Our Italics) This definition avoids tying pain to the stimulus. Activity induced in the nociceptor and nociceptive pathways by a noxious stimulus is not pain, which is always a psychological state, even though we may well appreciate that pain most often has a proximate physical cause.

These descriptions and definitions make it clear that the pain is not merely a response to an external stimulus. Rather, it is clearly a subjective psychological state, and as such, is influenced by much more than the associated physical stimulus.

Two contrasting examples may be helpful in visualizing the wide range of pain responses presented clinically by dental patients.

First is Karen, a 22-year-old student who is caries free but has localized gingivitis because of poor hygiene in some areas of her mouth. She reports the sensation of the rubber prophylaxis cup on her teeth as unbearable pain.

The second example is Richard, a 35-year-old construction worker, who often experiences bruises and other minor injuries at work. He was seen for a periodontal abscess. He had avoided treatment because he thought the swelling might be cancer. The area was anesthetized and debrided. Repeatedly during the procedure he tensed and screwed up the muscles of his face and brought his hands up as if in pain. However, when questioned he said he only was anticipating.

THEORIES OF PAIN

There have been many theories of pain. Van Frey in 1894 (Melzack and Wall, 1965) presented an extremely influential *specificity* theory. Specific pain receptors, when stimulated, were believed to result in pain. A one-to-one relationship was hypothesized between stimulation of nerve endings and the sensation of pain. Though alternative theories in which impulses were coded or patterned at the periphery and then modulated during transmission by central nervous system inputs existed as early as 1894, the specificity theory was most influential. Medical and dental texts considered pain in those terms. Detailed reviews of pain can be found in Clark and Hunt (1971), Melzack (1968), and Melzack and Wall (1965).

In the last three decades, there has been evidence that the specificity theory is insufficient to account for the phenomenon of clinical pain. Hill and associates (1952) showed that reduction of experimentally induced anxiety in subjects in laboratory experiments resulted in lowered intensity of pain. They have also shown that morphine reduces pain if the anxiety level is high but has no effect if anxiety is low.

Similarly, Beecher (1959) has argued that it is not possible to equate laboratory pain with clinical pain. Although morphine can be extremely effective in reducing pain reactions in clinical situations, it cannot be distinguished from saline in diminishing laboratory pain. In the clinic, placebo pain medications are effective in about one-third of the uses, but in the laboratory this percentage is reduced to almost zero. The missing ingredients in the laboratory are the anxiety and upset of the patient. Reducing pain in the clinic often involves reducing anxiety.

Beecher's classical (1959) study of soldiers also illustrates this point. Of 215 men studied who were seriously wounded in a battle, only 25 percent wanted a narcotic for relief. In comparison, over 80 percent of civilians with a similar surgical wound made under anesthesia requested narcotics. Beecher interpreted the difference in responses to the significance attributed to the wounds. In wartime, a battle wound meant relief, return to home alive, perhaps as a hero. In civilian life the surgery means disruption, cost, and disability. The setting influences the reaction to painful stimuli. Theorizing about pain must include such emotional and motivational factors.

One more bit of evidence: surgeons have attempted to use the knowledge gained in the laboratory to alleviate clinical pain by surgically severing branches of major facial nerves. This work, for example with atypical facial pain, produces unreliable results. Thus, the evidence for the success of cutting the nerve between the peripheral damage and the CNS gives little support for the specificity approach.

Laboratory study has focused on the sensory nature of pain. Pain receptors have been mapped, and neural pathways from peripheral to central areas have been established. However many such studies have excluded from investigation the psychological component of pain. Szasz (1957) theorized that laboratory studies have no relevance for clinical practice. The subjects know the pain will end soon and that no permanent tissue damage will occur. He concludes that the laboratory is not a useful place to examine pain responsivity, since it is impossible to arouse substantial anxiety in that setting. Dworkin and Chen (1982), twenty-five years later, have provided the first real experimental evidence that laboratory investigations may minimize pain responses. These researchers found that a clinical pain-producing dental situation yielded heightened pain and increased sensitivity compared with the pain experienced in a research laboratory using identical stimulation. The capacity of psychological variables, such as patient appraisal of threat, to lower pain thresholds cannot be overlooked. Findings from laboratory studies of anesthesia and pain that do not elicit anxiety may not generalize very well to clinical practice.

Melzack and Wall's (1965) gate control theory has been the most influential and important contemporary theory of pain perception. In short, their theory proposes that transmission of a noxious stimulus through a dorsal spinal gating mechanism is contingent upon not only the arrival of the stimuli, but also on other events in the periphery and on the set of the brain, which determines whether to permit the message to arrive. Three psychological processes were thought to contribute to perception of pain. These included the discrimination of sensory input, the subjective reaction to such input, and the cognitive evaluation of sensation. More than any other theoretical approach, gate control theory emphasizes the large role of psychological variables and how they affect the reaction to pain.

The gate control theory has been criticized because it does not account fully for all the neurophysiological data available today. The reader interested in greater detail is referred to Melzack and Wall (1965, 1970) and Melzack (1973).

Recently, Fordyce (1976), Sternbach and Fordyce (1975), and Gentry and Bernal (1977) have proposed that behavior, such as moaning, crying, distorted gait, or taking medication for pain relief, is an important component of pain. These researchers theorize that much of pain involves overt action and modification of this behavior is important in pain control.

FEAR AND PAIN

Before discussing the relationship of pain to fear, it is necessary to describe the theory of emotion and the importance of anticipation. The relationship between fear and pain is not simple. Some research shows that at an early stage, fear inhibits pain. Evidence exists that this inhibition occurs on the perceptual side, via descending pathways to interneurons in the dorsal horn of the spinal cord. This gating, mediated by endorphins and enkephalins, occurs at the first afferent synapse.

Endorphins and Pain Behavior

The recent research on opiate-like substances in brain tissue has promise of explaining the relationship between psychological and physiological functioning. Morphine-like agents, endorphins ("endorphin" is a contraction of "endogenous" and "morphine"), have been identified and are subjects of a variety of research—from biochemical to behavioral. Stressors, especially fear, are believed to trigger the release of endorphins from the pituitary resulting in an analgesic effect. As the stressor continues, naloxone, which antagonizes the analgesic, is released and pain is enhanced.

This is often the situation we face clinically. Those who are fearful in shorter restorative appointments do not show much upset; however, subsequent longer appointments are usually traumatic. Once fears are allayed, moreover, pain is much less likely to occur. Another indication that fear promotes pain is the widespread use of diazepam, sedative-hypnotics, and alcohol to treat and prevent pain. For many patients, 5–10 mg of diazepam or an ounce of alcohol are useful prior to dental treatment.

The principle is clear: *deal with the fear first,* and then pain will be a minor problem. But why should this occur? Fear is said to activate the endorphines; it should reduce pain induced by noxious stimuli. How can it sensitize the pain system? Bolles and Faneslow (1980), in their recent model of fear and pain, suggest muscle tension may be a factor. Anxiety produces muscle tension. This tension has a variety of physical effects including pain. Another complementary explanation is that it is not pain that causes the suffering patients report, but fear itself. The agony of a traumatic dental appointment may be due more to the fear than the pain. Patients may report the experience as painful because they can identify a fearful stimulus. The distress is not caused by the stimulus, i.e., the drilling activated pain. Rather, it is caused by mislabeling of the distress, such as being confined to a frightening situation. The mislabeling is hypothesized to arise from the fact that patient attention is focused, because of expectation, on the fearful stimulus. We have all learned that such a predicament—the inability to fight or flee—is painful. However, the dominant motivational system as discussed in Chapter 2 is fear, not pain.

Psychologists have presented other theories of the relationship between pain and fear. As we discussed in Chapter 2, the theories emphasize the conditioning of fear to stimuli sensed or thought of as painful. Clinically and experimentally, it is well established that when patients are anxious, they have a "lower pain threshold." In fact, all autonomic activation, not only fear, causes lower thresholds for pain and lower pain tolerance. The example of the athlete who feels no pain until the game is over is a clear example. Anticipation prior to the dental treatment itself has an effect upon pain threshold and tolerance. Patients who experience prolonged anticipatory arousal, usually with some form of catastrophic thought, are often not able to control themselves during the dental appointment. This arousal usually makes itself felt hours or even days prior to the appointment and elicits additional fear. Now the patient not only fears dental treatment, but also the aversiveness of his own arousal and its accompanying thoughts. Such situations often result in the patient being overwhelmed; his perceived lack of control—an inability to respond with desired fight or flight—contributes to the problem. This patient becomes panicky and looks physically drained. He may flee the dental chair in tears prior to treatment, avert the head during injection, or bite the dentist's finger. He may report nausea, shortness of breath, or dizziness. He may perspire profusely.

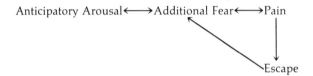

Note the arrows that go in both directions: Arousal causes additional fear, and additional fear enhances future fear and arousal. Pain not only leads to escape, but also to additional future fear and arousal. Effective management of the patient focuses efforts not only on in-chair anxiety but also on the anticipatory arousal and its labeling.

CULTURAL FACTORS AND PAIN

In this section we discuss how cultural factors influence pain and anxiety. Differences in the reactions to pain between individuals from different cultural backgrounds have received considerable study. It is apparent that cultural training has a major influence on reactions to painful stimuli. In 1952, Zbrowski's now classic work *People in Pain* called attention to the different ways in which cultural groups perceived and responded to pain. Jewish and Italian patients responded more emotionally to pain and tended to magnify it; "Old Americans" were more stoic, Irish patients were found to tend to deny pain. Since then, many scholarly papers have been presented on this subject. Blacks, Eskimos, American Indians, Puerto Ricans, and other ethnic and racial groups have been studied. Weisenberg (1977) reviewed these studies and placed them in a theoretical framework.

According to Weisenberg, major differences between cultural groups seem to be related to pain tolerance (the extent of noxious stimuli) rather than the threshold discrimination (initial level reported as pain) of pain as a sensation. Underlying attitude differences and reactions to anxiety appear to be a major source of these differences in pain tolerance. Weisenberg's comments:

> When outside sensory means for evaulation are reduced, the individual turns toward his social environment for validation of his judgments. Since pain is a private, ambiguous situation, comparison with others helps to determine what reactions are appropriate. Is it permissible to cry? Does one have to grin and bear it? When is it permissible to ask for help? . . .

People learn many of their anxieties and reactions by observing others. This process takes place in childhood, within families, as well as in social settings. For example, Craig and Best (1977) have shown that pain tolerance is subject to the social influence of models in a laboratory setting. Shoben and Borland (1954) have shown that experiences and attitudes of family members are very important in determining the individual's reaction to dental treatment. Similarly, Johnson and Baldwin (1968) found that children whose mothers had high anxiety scores showed more anxious behavior than children of mothers with low anxiety.

A few more points about the influence of cultural factors and pain need to be raised. Some findings ("myths" as Zbrowski called them in 1952) are based on very few observations in situations where the reactions of subjects may have been biased by the testing situation itself. For example, initial research by white researchers on pain tolerance of southern U.S. blacks predicted low pain tolerance (Katz, 1964). However, more recent studies report no difference between black and white obstetrical patients (Weisenberg, 1977) and medical students (Merskey and Spear, 1964). More importantly, these are generalizations that are often not predictive in use with the individual patient in the dental setting.

COPING WITH ANXIETY AND PAIN

How the patient ordinarily copes with stressful events may be important in developing an optimal dental pain control strategy. A few dimensions have been identified as being important and can be readily assessed.

Can the patient respond to stressors in his life with some sort of conscious *coping strategy*, or does the patient respond only with *catastrophizing* thoughts? Chaves and Brown (1978) interviewed a series of patients undergoing dental treatment. From this interview, patients were classified as to whether or not a coping strategy was used to reduce stress, and if not, whether catastrophizing thoughts were evident. They found those patients having some form of their own cognitive coping strategy experienced less stress than patients whose cognitive activity was characterized as catastrophizing. Similarly, in 1974, Chaves and Barber reported that the greater the amount of time subjects used either the researchers' cognitive strategy or their own strategy the greater the pain reduction in an experimental study.

It is our experience that some intensely fearful patients do not feel they have the ability to generate a pain coping strategy. This may not be necessary. Chaves and Brown (1974) found that it may be more important to avoid catastrophizing than to engage in positive coping. Clinically, identification and elimination of catastrophic ideations is always our first priority. Catastrophizing is much worse than not being able to generate a strategy.

In both Chaves and Brown's works and the recent study of Richardson and Kleinknecht (1984), catastrophizers were found to rate their dental procedures as more stressful than copers. Clearly, as noted earlier in this chapter, the stressfulness and pain of the dental experience are magnified by those who tend to show catastrophizing ideation.

Examples of Coping Strategies

Just like placid thoughts, pictures . . . I let my mind wander. Just think on different things like I look around and observe things in the room and let them bring my attention to them rather than what's going on in my mouth.

Well, I just tried basically in a philosophic way not to identify with the body. . . . Well, basically I was thinking of a mantra while it was taking place. To just negate is not enough—you have to have something to engage the mind also. So I was trying to get the mind not to think about what was going on in the body. . . .

I just try and prepare myself. You know it's going to hurt so I tell myself: "Just be ready for it—think about something else." And I tense up more or less when he puts it in and then I just relax and that's about it. (Adapted from Chaves and Brown, 1974)

A recent psychological inventory developed by Billings and Moos (1981) and illustrated below presents a profile of how an individual copes with stressful events. In this inventory, the patient identifies a recent personal crisis or stressful life event, e.g., the loss of a job, and then answers 19 yes/no questions that probe how he or she dealt with the event. Examples are "Tried to see positive side" or "Talked with a friend about the situation." The items are grouped into three methods of coping categories: active-cognitive, active-behavioral, and avoidance. The items are also classified into two foci of coping categories (problem-focused and emotion-focused). The score for each coping measure is the percentage of items answered "Yes." These measures of coping were found to influence how stress actually affected men and women and can be used clinically for deciding on a treatment strategy. (See Folkman and Lazarus, 1980 and Lazarus, 1980 for other studies of this phenomenon.)

The way this information could be used clinically is as follows:

1. Ask the patient to recall an earlier stressful event in his life and answer the questions on the inventory.

2. Discuss the results with the patient and suggest how he successfully dealt with another stressful event might be useful and transferable to the dental situation.

3. If the previous attempt was unsuccessful in the patient's mind, use these items to generate a discussion of other coping mechanisms available.

THE INFLUENCE OF PERSONALITY

Many personality traits of normal individuals have been associated with reactions to pain. A review of the literature yields conflicting results. The different definitions of personality make comparisons between studies hazardous. Moreover, most studies evaluate long-term chronic pain and its determinants. Acute pain, whether pathologic, e.g., toothache or abscess, or iatrogenic—injection or drilling—is the kind of pain we refer to when we think of going to the dentist. Reactions to acute and chronic pain are different (Sternbach, 1968; Fordyce, 1976).

Sensitizers versus Repressors

This dimension of personality focuses on styles of handling information. Does the patient try to cope by actively trying to deal with the stressor or does he try to reduce input? Individuals who welcome information, enjoy explanations of diagnostic and treatment procedures, desire to view the treatment, may be labeled as monitors or "sensitizers." Those who eschew information and are upset by knowing what is going on may be labeled "repressors" or blunters. There is evidence that they show different patterns of pre- and post-operative anxiety and respond, as you would predict, differently to information (DeLong, 1970). Pain responses also seem to be different (Neufeld and Davidson, 1971). Knowledge of where the patient lies on the sensitization-repression (monitor-blunter) continuum is useful in developing a successful strategy. Would information and explanation be very useful for a repressor? Or would a sensitizer like to listen to music? Hardly.

74

Locus of Control

This dimension of personality, which focuses on beliefs, has been widely studied. Briefly, locus of control is a belief regarding the degree to which people see themselves as being in control and responsible for what happens to them. A person with an "external" locus of control believes that whatever happens to him is a result of luck, fate, chance, powerful others, etc. For example, if he fails a test, it is because the test was unfair, the teacher inadequate, etc. The person with an "internal" locus of control believes that he is in control of what happens. If he fails a test, he believes that it was because he did not study sufficiently.

There is evidence that the scales that measure this personality dimension are useful predispositional measures. For example, Seeman and Evans (1962) found internal locus of control patients were better informed about their disease and asked more questions. Johnson et al. (1971) found internal locus of control surgical patients received more doses of analgesics than those exhibiting external locus of control. None of the dosages were extreme, and taking the analgesic can be interpreted as coping or adaptive. In fact, it appears that patients with external locus of control requested insufficient medication to control post-operative discomfort. Houston (1972) found that internals performed better on a task when given prior information that shock could be avoided contingent on their performance, whereas externals performed better when told that shock could not be avoided. Similarly, Auerbach et al. (1976) found internal subjects who viewed videotapes providing specific information about an imminent tooth extraction showed better adjustment during surgery than internals who viewed a general information tape about the clinic. Conversely, externals responded more favorably to the general information tape. A number of medical and dental studies, e.g., Duke and Cohen (1974) indicate that internals respond better to preventive and other recommendations that require active patient involvement; externals are believed to require more guidance and structuring. Examples from the 1966 version of Internal-External (I-E) scale, developed by Julian Rotter, are presented below. Patients are instructed to choose either "a" or "b" for each item.

1. a. Children get into trouble because their parents punish them too much.

   b. The trouble with most children nowadays is that their parents are too easy with them.

2. a. Many of the unhappy things in people's lives are partly due to bad luck.

   b. People's misfortunes result from the mistakes they make.

This scale can be used clinically to better understand a patient who can't describe clearly how much responsibility for his own care he will take. For example, will the patient practice relaxation exercises at home? Or follow oral self-care instructions?

Though belief in the efficacy of one's actions is an important personality dimension to be assessed, other aspects of control, independent of personality, are important. As suggested in Chapter 2, many patients who generally are in control of their lives feel vulnerable, unable to control the perceived danger of a dental appointment. Most of us prefer to have at least some control over an aversive event, and there is evidence that control over the pain situation can reduce stress and pain reactions. More about the issue of control may be found in Chapters 6–9.

Suggestibility

Research that seeks personality correlates of both waking and hypnotic suggestibility have not been very successful, although there are some useful results. Children between the ages of 7 and 14 have been found to be significantly more suggestible than adults (Barber and Calverley, 1963) possibly because children are usually quite dependent on others. Consequently, it may be easier to establish rapport, and then trust, with them than with adults. Some investigators have found significant correlations between dependency and suggestibility. Similarly, there is recent evidence that individuals who are more trusting are more suggestible (Periera and Austrin, 1980). Also, a silent, passive demeanor has been found to be helpful (Reyher et al., 1979). Suggestible subjects are less vigilant, restrict attention in peripheral visual fields, and are less responsive to auditory stimuli (Smyth, 1981).

Researchers have found that suggestibility is primarily situationally determined. That is, it is strongly influenced by the patients' expectations and the relationship with the clinician. Here, clinician characteristics may be important. Patient confidence in clinical personnel is important. Though prestige and technical competence may contribute to patient suggestibility, there is evidence that the status of the title of "doctor" or "dentist" may not be sufficient. Warmth may be more important (Smyth, 1981). Gryll and Katahn (1978) found that the pain of injection was influenced by the personal warmth of the clinician and confidence of the dentist in controlling pain.

There are simple behavioral tests that help to determine the degree to which the patient is, at any moment, susceptible to suggestion. One quick and easy test, described in detail in Chapter 9 in our discussion of using hypnosis clinically, involves suggesting that there is anesthesia in the patient's foot, hand, or lip.

CONTROLLING PAIN

Local Anesthetics

Local anesthetic drugs are of great importance in pain control. They are a key modality in ensuring a pain-free and relatively comfortable experience for the fearful patient. Surprisingly, few clinicians have a complete understanding of the effect of these potent drugs.

This section will review the basic mechanism and characteristics of local anesthetics and then discuss clinical problems encountered with fearful patients: anesthetic failure and adverse effects. It is beyond the scope of this text to teach local anesthetic technique. Readers are referred to S. F. Malamed, *Handbook of Local Anesthesia* (St. Louis: Mosby Co., 1980) and similar texts for more complete information.

Susan, a 35-year-old school teacher, was referred to us, in part, because she could not become numb enough to tolerate a crown preparation on tooth #31. Our findings suggest that the dentist used too little anesthetic, waited too long for anesthesia onset, and inappropriately withdrew the vasoconstrictor. After managing Susan's fear, she was anesthetized successfully and the crown completed.

The injectable local anesthetics were introduced early in the 20th century. Procaine (Novocaine®) was the first practical drug and although it was thought likely to produce allergic responses, it remained in use until the late 1940's. Lidocaine, introduced in 1948, has become the most commonly used dental anesthetic drug. It produces more dependable pulpal and soft tissue anesthesia than procaine and has low allergic potential.

Other drugs, such as mepivacaine and prilocaine, were introduced later and have been reported to have longer duration without vasoconstrictors. Otherwise, their mechanism of action is similar to that of lidocaine.

The newer drugs are classified as amides because of their chemical structure. Procaine is an ester-type anesthetic. The anesthetics work by crossing neuronal membranes and acting on the inner surface of the axonal membrane, blocking both generation and conduction of nerve impulses.

Drug Formulations

In the United States, dental anesthetics are primarily sold in 1.8-ml glass carpules (2.2 ml in Great Britain) containing anesthetic agent, preservative (usually paraben*), and a vasoconstrictor. Nearly all the drugs used in dentistry today are of the amide class. The key distinction between the drugs is length of action with the most common drugs (lidocaine, mepivacaine) being relatively medium acting, and less common drugs (e.g., bupivacaine, etidiocaine) being long acting. The duration depends on the drug

---

* Since 1981 manufacturers have begun removing paraben from local anesthetics because it may cause hypersensitivity. However, some drug formulations may still contain it.

TABLE 3-1
Amide Local Anesthetic Drugs

Chemical Name	Representative Brand Names	Relative Duration
Lidocaine	Xylocaine®	Medium
Mepivacaine	Carbocaine®	Medium
Prilocaine	Citanest®	Medium
Bupivacaine	Marcaine®	Long

itself, the vasoconstrictor, and site of injection. Table 3-1 lists the drugs commonly used in dentistry.

DOSAGE. It is not known exactly how much anesthetic is generally given in dental practice. It is likely that one or two 1.8-ml carpules of medium duration drugs are routinely given. These dosages are far below the maximum safe dosage levels and may account for many reports of inadequate anesthesia.

The maximum dosages for local anesthetic drugs (Accepted Dental Therapeutics, 1982) to be used in dental therapy are given in Table 3-2.

ONSET. Many of the fear reactions we have seen on referral in our clinic have been labeled by dentists as reactions to an anesthetic drug or vasoconstrictor. A good part of the problem is the long period many practitioners employ between injections, testing for anesthesia, and beginning actual operations. This is particularly true in the mandible where it is not uncommon for 15–20 minutes to elapse between the injection of a single carpule and another, often with the message by the dentist that the first "did not work." A major contributor to this is an inadequate quantity of anesthetic. As suggested above, one carpule is probably not adequate for reliable anesthesia for operative dentistry or endodontics in many areas of the mouth.

However, a major misconception is that anesthesia onset is very slow and that waiting 10–15 minutes helps. Since problems occur most often in the mandibular block regional injection, this is a good example. Research shows 90 percent of persons will have the onset of lip symptoms in 65–75

TABLE 3-2
Maximum Dosages for Local Anesthetic Drugs

Drug	Dose
Prilocaine	400 mg
Lidocaine	300 mg
Mepivacaine	300 mg
Bupivacaine	175 mg

seconds, with onset of long acting drugs being longer than medium drugs. Periosteal anesthesia was obtained in over 90 percent of cases in about 3 minutes.

We discuss injection technique again in Chapter 6; however, our clinical practice is to give a single carpule, wait about one minute for the onset of soft tissue symptoms and proceed "painlessly" to administer a full dose of the drug. This avoids the "aura" of anesthetic failure and the inevitable increase in patient anxiety associated with the anticipation that "I might get hurt. . . ."

AREA OF ANESTHESIA. For reasons that are not clear, some dentists with whom we have worked developed a habit of not anesthetizing a large enough area to work painlessly. This is particularly true for the palate where the injections are perceived by the dentist to be painful. The dentist's reluctance is picked up by the patient and often translated into requests to avoid these injections. Inevitably, however, this results in discomfort during the operative or periodontal procedure.

Problem of Inadequate Local Anesthesia

Although pain control is considered a requisite of restorative dentistry, and local anesthesia is the method of choice for most patients in the United States and Canada, there are few studies of its success. Textbooks recommend a variety of clinical techniques and are not very consistent in their discussions of success rates. Clinical "failures" are reported to result from very short duration of anesthesia, injection technique, the properties of the anesthetic agent, unusual nerve anatomy, or infection. Malamed, in the *Handbook of Local Anesthesia,* reports successful mandibular block in 80–97 percent of injections, depending on the technique employed. He believes failures are attributable to the density of the mandible, limited accessibility of the nerves, and anatomical variation. He reports a success rate of 95 percent in maxillary injections. He attributes the high success rate to less dense bone and easy accessibility but does not hypothesize a reason for failures. The usual criteria for anesthesia is sufficient numbness to allow tooth preparation without pain (pulpal anesthesia).

There are two basic types of studies: (1) reports of clinical observations and (2) laboratory studies. Clinical studies often report both the incidence of anesthetic failures and attribute causation. Laboratory studies, in both animals and humans, most often evaluate the dosage-duration relationship for anesthetics and do not address anesthetic failures.

These studies are reviewed in detail by Kaufman, Weinstein, and Milgrom (1984). Though there are many dental and non-dental reports of the relationship between fear and pain, the literature is generally silent on psychological factors that may influence inadequate anesthesia. Factors such as fear are clearly capable of influencing patient response to painful or other stimuli applied after administration of local anesthetic. As such, these factors may contribute to inadequate anesthesia. Moreover, the relationship between these variables may be reciprocal: fear leading to inadequate anesthesia and being treated with inadequate anesthesia serves to increase fear.

To begin to evaluate the extent of problems with local anesthetics in clinical practice, 200 Washington State general dentists were randomly selected from the Washington State Dental Association directory and surveyed. Dentists reported inadequate anesthesia, on average, for 13 percent of all patients even in the previous five days. The vast majority of dentists reported some inadequate anesthesia. Years of practice experience did not influence the rate; practical experience itself did not lead to more successful pain control.

Rates for inadequate anesthesia differed by type of injection. Man-

81

dibular blocks presented the greatest problem, followed by maxillary posterior and maxillary anterior injections. In response to initial anesthetic failure, almost all dentists gave an additional injection. However, disrupted or lengthened visits were extremely common. Dentists also indicated that high percentages (47 percent) of patients were fearful or anxious.

Improving Anesthesia

There are steps that can be taken to reduce failures and enhance the grade of anesthesia. First, the dentist should prepare patients for local anesthesia injection. Does the patient have a history of anesthetic failure? Research has shown that relaxed patients are able to achieve greater pain control than those who are tense (Bobey and Davidson, 1970). We recommend that the dental staff observe the patient carefully before treatment begins. Is respiration and heart rate slow and rhythmic? Or, is breathing quickened and the pulse racing? Are muscles relaxed or tense? The face and hands should be watched. Most patients are able to relax sufficiently by taking a few short breaths, concentrating on exhalation. This breathing exercise might be accompanied by the suggestion that it will lead to relaxation and greater comfort during dental procedures. Trust and rapport are essential if this procedure is to be effective. For extremely tense patients, relaxation procedures, hypnosis, or biofeedback in conjunction with relaxation, are effective. Dentists who employ N_2O/O_2 will find these approaches can be used both before and during inhalation sedation and will enhance the result. This is also true for dentists who use premedication or IV medications.

Second, the dentist should review and perfect his or her techniques of administering local anesthesia. The topical anesthesia should be used to give the patient the feeling of numbness. Often, we find it helpful to place it first on the tongue to teach the patient the sensation. Then when it is placed on the gingiva, the patient will be better able to feel its effect. Many times it is helpful to ask the patient to affirm feeling the anesthetic effect of the topical before proceeding. Then, the local anesthetic should be injected slowly to minimize discomfort. During the injection it is helpful to suggest to the patient the sensation of numbness spreading and becoming more complete. Use adequate volumes of anesthetic and if the onset of anesthesia is not forthcoming in a minute or so, an additional injection should be administered. Prolonging this time interval is inefficient and does not contribute to a better result. Patients with anesthetic failure histories should be given larger doses initially.

Finally, drilling is the only true test of dental anesthesia we have; and as such, some small number of patients will report pain even when they are relaxed. Painless drilling is one of the miracles of modern dentistry, and under most circumstances, treatment should not proceed if the patient is reporting discomfort. Most often these patients have subjective signs of soft tissue anesthesia. However this does not necessarily indicate the presence of pulpal anesthesia. Our experience with patients with long histories of anesthetic failure is that if we employ appropriate relaxation procedures, then supplementary injections (such as the intraligamentary) are effective. However, we find it is important for the dentist to remain especially objective at this stage. If anesthesia remains inadequate, then perhaps infection or some other biological cause is at work.

In situations where repeated injections result in failure, a sedative filling may be placed. We find patients are able to accept biological explanations for anesthetic failure and are relieved to know the dentist does not think they are "crazy." Before the next appointment, the dentist should review the pain control procedures to be employed. We find oral premedication or additional relaxation exercises to practice at home help reduce the anxiety associated with the anesthetic injection. Also, collateral nerve supply should be carefully considered and supplementary injections given initially. The dentist should create the expectation in the patient that a stronger, more effective drug is being used now. In our experience, under these circumstances, anesthesia will be effective and the dentist's reputation as well as patient comfort enhanced.

The following case history provides an illustration of the application of the above principles.

John, a 30-year-old construction worker, came to our clinic after avoiding dental care for the past 13 years. He reported that as an adult he had difficulty getting numb. "Novocaine doesn't work on me. The last time I was injected eleven times with the needle." He reported additional accounts of multiple injections without the desired effect. "The pain was always unbearable; the injections don't do their job for me."

John was given relaxation instructions and practiced deep breathing in the chair prior to treatment. During the intial interview it was learned that he was an avid fisherman. This information was utilized in hypnosis and relaxation was achieved. After the topical anesthetic was applied, two carpules of "special anesthetic" (2% lidocaine with 1:100,000 epinephrine) were injected to anesthetize tooth #5. The decay was deep and the patient reported minor sensitivity in the pulpal wall area while it was being removed. Instead of reinjecting, which might not have been successful and would have reinforced the patient's expectation that he could not be numb, the dentist placed a sedative filling. The next week the restoration was completed. The patient reported no discomfort at any of five subsequent restorative appointments. Moreover, at the last appointment, he fell asleep in the chair! Pushing ahead to finish the restoration at the initial appointment would have resulted in a clinical failure.

Long Acting Anesthetics

Earlier in this chapter we suggested that some anesthetics available to dentists (e.g., bupivacaine) have relatively longer duration than the more common lidocaine. Advocates for these drugs initially argued that they would reduce post-operative analgesic use after surgery. Results of such studies were disappointing, and little clinical difference emerged. However, the drugs appear to be useful in certain emergency situations. When a patient is in pain from an endodontically involved tooth, anesthesia adequate for pulp treatments is difficult to achieve. This is especially true if the patient has been in pain for a while and is tired and sleepless. As an alternative to proceeding immediately, we recommend an injection of bupivacaine and prescription of oral analgesics (and antibiotics if necessary). After the patient has rested and become calmer, the anxiety will have been reduced and it will be easier and more successful to proceed with normal local anesthetic and endodontic procedures. This procedure is especially useful if the emergency call comes at night or on a weekend.

Problem of Adverse Effects

Before discussing adverse effects, a definition is necessary. Evers and Haegerstam (1981) define an adverse effect as an untoward reaction to the administration of local anesthetics including allergic reactions, systemic toxic reactions, psychogenic effects, or drug interactions.

The frequency of adverse effects reported in dentistry is much higher than in medicine. Adverse effects range to 30 percent of the appointments in which anesthetics are administered. They also differ in type. In medicine they are mostly toxic. In dentistry they appear to be somatic manifestations of fear, which we believe may or may not occur with a cognitive component. Effects include palpitations, dizziness, nausea, tremor, sweating, pallor, and fainting. Interestingly, these effects are similar to systemic reaction to intravenous vasoconstrictor administration. Persson (1969) postulates that adverse effects appearing within 1–2 minutes of injection are likely due to the body's own release of epinephrine rather than to the effects of local anesthetic or vasoconstrictor, although evidence is lacking.

Two large clinically based dentistry studies have been reported in which local anesthetic reactions have been evaluated. In one double-blinded study (Goldman and Gray, 1963) 67 dentists in four different dental settings (hospital, military, dental school, and private practice) reported 12,079 cases involving the use of 3% prilocaine with epinephrine 1:300,000, 2% prilocaine with 1:200,000 epinephrine, and 2% lidocaine with 1:80,000 epinephrine. The overall frequency of side effects was 11.4 percent, a percentage the investigators found unexpectedly high.

In another, more controlled double-blind study in which data were collected over a 10-month period, patients received local anesthetics with and without vasoconstrictors (Persson, 1969). The investigator recorded adverse effects in 75 of 2960 cases (2.5 percent). The reports included pallor, nausea, sweating, dizziness, and fainting. The author was unable to associate increased concentrations of vasoconstrictors with increased adverse effects. Similar findings were reported by Moose (1959). On the other hand, one study showed an increased percentage of adverse effects with 2% procaine with 1:50,000 epinephrine versus 2% procaine alone for dental student subjects (Costich, 1956).

Evaluation of topical anesthetics has been minimal. Topical anesthetics are administered in order to reduce the pain associated with needle insertion. Theoretically they could reduce adverse effects of the anesthetic caused by anxiety. Improper applications, however, may make their use ineffective. Rate of onset of anesthesia takes from 2–5 minutes, much slower than anesthesia by injection (ADT, 1982). If the procedure is hurried, a resulting painful injection may lead to fear. Many of the preparations are ester-type anesthetics that may cause an allergic reaction. Moreover, some preparations are marketed in pressurized spray containers that are difficult to control, either in dose or site of application. Pollack (1966) postulates that suggestion rather than the topical anesthetic, itself, may be the critical factor in determining whether the patient feels the placement of the anesthetic needle. Among the subjects receiving topical anesthetic, nearly 69 percent of those told it would not hurt reacted indifferently to the injection, whereas only 58 percent of those receiving no suggestion remained calm. Moreover, when extreme patient reactions did occur, they happened nearly twice as frequently in the control group (6.4 percent) as in the experimental groups (3.7 percent). Results of studies involving topical anesthetics may be difficult to interpret due to the potential presence of adverse effects associated with the local anesthetic or the injection procedure itself.

Patient Factors

Evidence exists in the literature to suggest that patient characteristics influence local anesthetic adverse effects. Factors hypothesized include fear, prior experience associated with local anesthetics (including being treated without being numb), misattribution of drug effects, medical conditions and drug interactions, drug history, and age (related to fear) and sex.

FEAR. Fear of the dentist appears to be widespread. Scott and Hirschman (1982) estimate that between 22–79 percent of the population may be at least somewhat dentally anxious, whereas 8–15 percent may be highly anxious. Other estimates fall within this range as well (Agras, 1969; Freidsen and Feldman, 1958). At the University of Washington Dental Fear Research Clinic, patients were assessed for fear prior to treatment and again after completion of a series of six to ten dental treatment visits. Average scores for the categories "Seeing the anesthetic needle" and "Feeling the needle injected" were nearly 25 percent lower at post-treatment re-test in a series of 20 patients (Smith et al., 1984). Shannon and Isbell (1963) have demonstrated elevated levels of epinephrine (as indicated by serum levels of corticosteroids) during injection. Three groups of subjects were injected with different solutions (lidocaine, lidocaine with epinephrine 1:100,000, saline), a fourth underwent needle insertions with no injection, and a fifth sham group went through the anesthetic procedure without needle insertion. All groups were found to have similar elevated levels of circulating corticosteroids. These results suggest psychological factors to be important variables during injections.

The foregoing discussion suggests that the injection procedure is fear-producing for some individuals and that fear can influence endogenous epinephrine release resulting in symptoms such as tachycardia, heart palpitations, syncope, sweating, and other cardiovascular effects.

PRIOR EXPERIENCE. Some evidence exists to suggest that a patient's history with local anesthetic may be predictive of future adverse effects. Persson (1969) noted that 1 percent (30/2960) of his subjects had "on more than one occasion previously experienced general side reactions to local anesthetic." Of this total, 40 percent subsequently reported at least one adverse effect during the course of the study. Goldman and Gray (1963) reported 5 percent of 12,079 cases had a history of adverse effects. The effects were not enumerated. Another example of previous experience with local anesthetic involves patients being treated without profound anesthesia. Persson (1969) found 14 percent (372/2960) of his cases with adverse effects to have had only partial or unsuccessful anesthesia. Partial anesthesia was defined as some pain during procedure not requiring a supplementary dose of anesthetic. Unsuccessful anesthesia required 1 or more supplementary doses. The overall percentage of adverse effects with complete anesthesia was 2 percent (57/2558). However partial anesthesia resulted in 4 percent (14/318) having side effects and unsuccessful anesthesia 7 percent (4/54). It is unknown if being treated while not numb was considered to be a previous adverse reaction to local anesthetic in this study. Nor is it known how many of the 372 reporting incomplete anesthesia had a prior history of failure to get numb. In a recent survey of an insured dental population (Weinstein et al., in press), 60 percent of subjects reporting anesthetic failure at their last dental visit also reported previous difficulty in getting numb. Kaufmann et al. (1984) reported a high percentage of dental anxiety (47 percent) among patients with a history of failure to get numb. Milgrom et al. (1984) suggest this anxiety may lead to further anesthetic failure resulting in mismanagement by the dentist and inappropriate use of local anesthetics. This in turn may lead to further adverse effects.

MISATTRIBUTION. The reported incidence of true local anesthetic allergies is extremely low (VanArsdel, 1984). Nonetheless, patients are frequently advised that adverse reactions experienced during injections are allergic in nature and particular anesthetic solutions should be avoided. DeShazo and Nelson (1979) allergy tested 90 patients referred with the diagnosis of lidocaine allergy, including 14 having a history of immediate hypersensitivity reaction. Not one of the 90 proved hypersensitive when skin tested and challenged with increasing concentrations of the drug. In a similar study, Babajews and Ivanyi (1982) found only 3 patients out of 37 reporting previous untoward reactions to be allergic. Aldrete and Johnson (1970) surveyed 809 incidents of drug reaction. Allergies were found in 525 cases, but local anesthetic could be implicated only three times. Other drugs with frequent adverse reactions are also subject to allergy mislabeling. Allergic rashes associated with ampicillin constitute only 1/3 of the rashes seen accompanying this drug (Geyman and Erickson, 1978). Yet patients are frequently taken off the drug unnecessarily and advised to avoid ampicillin and other penicillins in the future. Moreover, VanArsdel (1982) reports that patients with known penicillin allergies can frequently be treated successfully with the drug within two years of their last reaction. He estimates that five out of six individuals with positive testing of penicillin allergy can safely receive the antibiotic.

Mislabeling of adverse drug reactions may lead to more expensive and/or less effective treatment alternatives. For example, Malamed (1973) has recommended diphenhydramine as a substitute for individuals reported allergic to local anesthetics. This antihistamine, however, is known to be less effective as a local anesthetic in duration and quality of anesthesia and may cause pain during injection. This may lead to elevated fear levels and increased adverse effects. Other alternatives such as general anesthesia or IV sedation may prove unacceptable due to cost or increased medical risk, leading to avoidance of treatment and worsening of dental problems. In short, due to misunderstanding or lack of knowing the cause of local anesthetic adverse effects, dentists themselves may be contributing to the increased frequency of untoward effects.

MEDICAL HISTORY. Concurrent medical problems may enhance the chances of local anesthetic adverse effects either through the emotional state of the individual or through medications being taken to counteract the condition. Individuals with a history of other allergies may manifest allergic reactions to local anesthetic or other therapeutic agents used in dentistry (ADT, 1982). Patients suffering from chronic respiratory disease may be in respiratory acidosis and have elevated blood levels of epinephrine. As a result, they may be more prone to develop syncope, tachycardia, sweating, tremors, or palpitations on administrations of even low doses of anesthetics with vasoconstrictors. Hypertensive and uncontrolled thyroid conditions may also cause untoward effects in the presence of exogenous doses of vasoconstrictors (Jastek, 1983). Hypochondriacal patients (Brown and Vaillant, 1981) may find difficulty coping with stressful events such as going to the dentist. Some may even find these events so catastrophic as to fear major consequences, such as death, as a result of a dental visit (Smith et al., 1984). Finally, some of these individuals may presently be taking antidepressants, phenothiazines, beta-blocking drugs, adrenergic neuron blocking agents, or thyroid hormones, all of which are known to interact with vasoconstrictors (Jastek, 1983).

Dentist Variables

Dentist variables relate to what the dentist does during injections based upon his/her beliefs, knowledge, and experience. It is important to consider communication with the patient, length of injection time, use of aspirating syringes, and drug knowledge.

Studies of dental fear have shown that dentist behavior and communications skills are important etiologic factors (Smith et al., 1984). Providing clear explanations, taking adequate time so the patient does not feel rushed, listening to patient concerns, and credibility of what the dentist says have been shown to reduce pain (Dangott et al., 1978) and may influence the incidence of local anesthetic adverse effects. Injecting too rapidly may cause pain and elevate fear levels. Moreover, apprehension may increase with prolonged waiting time between injections when supplemental doses are required. Kaufman et al. (1984) suggest increased volumes of anesthetics be used at the outset, with supplementary doses to follow if signs of anesthesia do not appear within one to two minutes. The use of aspirating syringes has been recommended by the Council on Dental Materials and Devices who note that positive aspirations of blood were reported among 2.6–30 percent of inferior alveolar injections in different series of patients (Alling and Christopher, 1974). A positive aspiration means either that the point of the needle is in a vessel or in a pool of blood. Failure to move the needle away from this area may lead to intravascular injections and toxicity. Traeger (1979) suggests that a hematoma resulting from such an accident may provide one reason for anesthetic failures, particularly within the inferior alveolar nerve site. In addition, Oikarinen et al. (1975) demonstrated that needle gauge is an unimportant factor in eliciting pain during injections.

Experience (i.e., years since graduation) did not appear to influence the rate of anesthetic failures in a survey of 93 dentists in Washington State (Kaufman et al., 1984). However, a lack of knowledge of local anesthetics may well lead to adverse effects if the dentist changes drugs during a treatment visit after failing to achieve anesthesia the first time. Use of an anesthetic without a vasoconstrictor may assure inadequate anesthesia and increase the chances of adverse effects, especially if work is attempted with resulting pain (Milgrom et al., 1984b). Bernstein et al. (1979) have shown that the most highly feared aspects of dentistry are painful dental procedures.

Dentists' beliefs concerning local anesthetics may be a function of early training in dental school. There the student is taught very little about either the recognition of systematic fear or its treatment (Milgrom et al., 1984). Fiset and Weinstein (1983) have demonstrated that dentists may not attend to all verbal and non-verbal indications of distress. Therefore, local adverse effects may be misattributed to the drug rather than to some other factor relating to the patients themselves, resulting in misuse of drugs and mismanagement of the patients, which may lead to further adverse effects.

In all, the literature shows that the dentist is an important factor in the etiology of fear, which may be a potent risk factor in the incident of local anesthetic adverse effects. Appropriate behavior and a thorough knowledge of local anesthetics as well as an ability to diagnose psychogenic side effects may prove beneficial in the overall reductions of these untoward events.

Patient Physiology

A large body of experimental data supports the idea that fear responses in human beings may be triggered by beta-adrenergic agonists, and beta-blockers have been found to be useful clinically to control these responses. These responses appear to be very similar to the anesthetic effects that have been reported. Pitts and Allen (1982) cite considerable evidence that epinephrine injection produces anxiety symptoms in neurotic patients who show their specific symptom pattern with the injection. Though epinephrine has both alpha- and beta-adrenergic actions, the beta-adrenergic component has been identified as responsible. Frohlich et al. (1966) used isoproterenol infusion, a pure beta-adrenergic agonist with no alpha-adrenergic action, to stimulate anxiety symptoms and anxiety attacks among anxious patients. Normal controls developed far fewer and less severe anxiety symptoms.

The mechanism of action of epinephrine infusion has been identified. According to Pitts and Allen (1982) epinephrine removes a calcium ion from the receptor site and initiates a series of biochemical steps that results in increased heart rate, constriction of splanchnic blood vessels, and dilation of blood vessels in major muscles, the skin, and the brain. Activation of the anaerobic glycolytic pathway results in increased lactate production from muscles and other tissues. They note that the effect of epinephrine infusion on blood pressure is highly variable. "The subject is always aware, however, of increased heart rate (palpitations) and physiologic changes that result in a variable degree of tension, tremulousness, apprehension and paresthesia. This severe anxiety-related phenomenon occurs with persons subject to anxiety experience and not with normal controls."

Lactate production itself has been found to be related to the somatic component of fear. Pitts and McClure (1962) found that an infusion of lactate and to a lesser extent lactate with calcium added, but not a glucose in saline control, would create somatic symptoms of anxiety for patients with anxiety neurosis but not for normals. This study was replicated by Fink et al. (1969).

The treatment of untoward reactions is to stop dental therapy and immediately administer palliative and supportive strategies. Vital signs should be monitored. Prevention always involves a careful history ruling out organic disease and allergy and an assessment of dental fear. Then both behavioral and pharmacological approaches are successful in reducing ill effects with injections at other appointments. Behavioral treatment involves the use of attribution and biofeedback (see Chapter 9). Pharmacologic treatment may involve the use of beta-blockers.

Ancillary Agents

This section focuses on the use of other antianxiety drugs and includes discussion of placebos. A number of drugs have been recommended for use in the control of dental anxiety, such as meprobamate, diazepam, the barbiturates, and nitrous oxide. While use of these agents is widespread (ADT, 1982), there are few data on even their general effectiveness with a dentally anxious population.

THE OLDER GROUPS OF ANXIOLYTIC AGENTS. These agents (meprobamate, chlordiazepoxide and the like) have not been shown to be useful with dental fear, especially in controlling physiologic components.

Most systems in the body are affected by fear. For example, in the cardio-vascular system fear increases systolic blood pressure, causes tachycardia, vasoconstriction of extremities and splanchnic regions and vasodilation in striated muscles, thus producing symptoms of palpitations, headaches, and cold fingers (Lader, 1983). Persson (1969) attempted to evaluate the effects of three common oral premedications (chlordiazepoxide, mepro-bamate, and prometazine) and a placebo during oral surgical procedures on a normal population. The calming effects of the drugs were to be measured by both behavioral ratings and urinary catecholamine excretion above basal levels. Drugs were administered one hour before surgery. Results indicated the drugs did not differ from one another in their influence on the excretion of catecholamines, nor appear to produce behavioral effects. Since the mean age of the subjects in this study ($n = 60$) was 19.4 years, a significant number may have been children. Dosages were age-dependent rather than weight-dependent, and a number of individuals may not have received adequate dosages. Moreover, catecholamines contained in the local anesthetic may have masked differences in the effect of premedication on the endogenous production of catecholamines. Finally, no data were provided to indicate the fear levels of patients receiving pre-medications prior to the surgical procedures. Thus, the results in this study remain inconclusive.

A similar study comparing meprobamate to placebo premedication was unable to detect differences on the cardiovascular system, i.e., blood pressure and heart rate (Persson, 1969). Other researchers (Berger, 1956, and Lundberg, 1959) had similar findings of the effects of meprobamate on the circulatory system.

BENZODIAZEPINES. These have recently become very popular with dentists. Specifically, diazepam is the most commonly used agent in dental practice for the treatment of anxiety or fear (Holt and Gaskins, 1982). It has a rapid onset of action and has been thought of as the drug of choice where this is a major consideration. As with the older anxiolytic agents, there have been few adequately designed medical or dental trials (Shader and Greenblatt, 1983). Though Holt and Gaskins (1982) note that "orally administered dosages have proven to be helpful in reducing anxiety associated with dental procedures," support for their statement is very meager. The regimen tested by Baird and Curson (1970)—5 mg at bedtime, 5 mg upon rising, and 5 mg two hours prior to the appointment—is frequently touted, although the conclusions provide little clinical guidance. The design in the study was weak, namely, lack of measurement or control of baseline anxiety, and the measures themselves were inadequate. Even though the drug reduced anxiety more than the placebo during an initial visit, there were no signficant differences between placebo and diazepam during the second treatment session and 39 of 100 patients were not able to discriminate between the two drugs. Thus, at best, the effects are highly unreliable. It should be noted that though relatively safe, benzodiazepines are not devoid of "hazards and side effects" (Hollister, 1975).

Overall, although antianxiety agents have a long history in dentistry as premedication, there are few data showing that they are very effective. Moreover, patients are notoriously unreliable pill-takers—unsupervised oral premedications are often not taken or taken incorrectly. On the other hand, the placebo value of these drugs appears to be substantial for patients who utilize drugs to assist in coping with stress.

Intravenous administration of diazepam is said to be preferred over the oral route (Holt and Gaskins, 1982). These authors note the following advantage: titration using exact increments, rapid achievement of desired pharmacological effects, an open line maintained via the continuous IV drip, and "ready acceptance of the procedure by apprehensive patients." This last point is not documented and is questionable. Many studies cite a variety of complications. Moreover, special training is required to use diazepam and other agents intravenously, and we believe they should be used primarily in in-patient facilities. There are situations for which IV diazepam is warranted. Patients who refuse to learn coping skills or who have many, very acute treatment needs may be candidates. Nonetheless, the use of such drugs is not without risk.

ORAL PREMEDICATION AND NITROUS OXIDE. As an alternative to IV drugs, oral premedication and nitrous oxide (N_2O) have been important for dentistry because of their ease and relative safety. The use of N_2O for conscious sedation has been increasing; it is estimated that it is used by about 25 percent of all practicing dentists in this country. Interviews concerning the pharmacological practice of a sample of Washington State dentists indicated even greater reliance on nitrous oxide.

A random sample of King County, Washington, general practitioners and pedodontists indicated that 32 of 35 dentists contacted (92 percent) used oral premedication on child patients, at least in selected cases. Of the 32 premedicating dentists, 26 (81 percent) used nitrous oxide. No difference was found between general practitioners and pedodontists for use of nitrous oxide or other premedications. It should be noted that the proportion of pedodontists now using nitrous oxide appears to be much greater (35 percent versus 93 percent) than that found in a 1971 survey of pedodontic diplomates (American Association of Pedodontic Diplomates, 1972) or in a larger study of pedodontists conducted by Wright and McAuley (1973). The second most frequent drug utilized was Valium® (13 percent). Practitioners reported a wide range in percentages of patients receiving premedication. Whereas 14 of the 32 dentists (43 percent) used premedication on less than 10 percent of their patients, 10 dentists (31 percent) used premedication in more than 80 percent of their patients. Premedication, especially nitrous oxide, appears to be a routine child management technique.

EFFECT OF NITROUS OXIDE OXYGEN. Although the use of nitrous oxide is perceived as an old and effective method for managing fear associated with dental visits, almost all research on the effect of this drug has dealt with its analgesic properties. These effects on children and adults have been clearly defined in a number of clinical and experimental studies conducted by Emmertsen (1965), Hogue, Ternisky, and Iranpour (1971), Berger (1972), and Devine et al. (1979). In all these studies, analgesic effects increased with increased gas concentration. Individual differences were considerable; however, wide variation from subject to subject was reported at the same concentration of nitrous oxide. Parallel findings are reported in a recent behavioral evaluation of nitrous oxide in Sweden. Reports of a recent study of 1719 treatment sessions in 823 patients, mainly of uncooperative children, indicate that behavioral responses to the drug—acceptance of the drug and treatment, treatment with difficulty, or non-acceptance of the drug and treatment—were highly variable both between and within patients (Hallonsten et al., 1983).

Nathan (1983) hypothesizes that this variation occurs because of the highly insoluble nature of N_2O in the blood, and rapid duration of onset, action, and elimination. Also, the mask delivery of N_2O constitutes an open air system highly subject to dilution with ambient air. Mouthbreathing, whether caused by habit, respiratory congestion, or emotional upset, reduces the effect of the drug. Continuous clinician titration of concentration to achieve desired effects while controlling undesirable side effects is needed.

Nathan notes that "it is conceivable that 10–20% N_2O may produce satisfactory sedation in one patient, whereas even 40–50% may be insufficient to elicit similar effects on another patient." On the other hand, experience with treating dental phobics at the University of Washington Dental Fears Research Clinic has shown that higher levels of nitrous oxide-oxygen sedation (50 percent +) are frequently less effective in controlling anxiety than are lower doses (20–30 percent) unrelated to the analgesic effect.

The ability of nitrous oxide to manage patient anxiety has not received as careful attention as the drug's analgesic effect. The few studies that exist, with the exception of the work of Nathan (1984) who compared N_2O, O_2, and an unmasked control group, are poor. This is extremely unfortunate, because the present approach in the clinical literature is to de-emphasize the analgesic effect of nitrous oxide exceeding 40 percent and to emphasize the sedative benefits of concentrations less than 40 percent. It should be noted that the professional literature recognizes that nitrous oxide sedation is only a helpful "aid" or "adjunct." Warnings are often proffered that nitrous oxide sedation is not a substitute for non-pharmacological patient management techniques. In other words, there is at least recognition that non-pharmacological considerations influence the effectiveness of the sedative technique. Dealing with fearfulness toward dental treatment should be a goal of treatment.

Although there are a few clinicians who utilize N_2O to manage all their patients, most clinicians utilize the drug selectively. However, empirical selection criteria for the use of N_2O have not been developed. The pedodontic literature discusses factors in drug selection. For example, Musselman and McClure (1975) note immediacy, extensiveness of treatment, and stress tolerance of the patient are important selection criteria. Preventive utilization of the drug also appears in the literature. For example, N_2O is often recommended for the tense but cooperative child or to help overcome brief but uncomfortable procedures such as injections and placements of rubber dam and clamps.

The clinical literature often explicitly states that the psychological preparation is important. Barenie's (1979) suggestions, which focus on the use of N_2O with children, are typical:

> More important than the physical preparation of the equipment is the psychologic preparation of the child and the introductory technic used. The child must understand that he will not be "put to sleep," but will be awake and aware at all times. The "Tell-Show-Do" approach is most helpful in establishing rapport with the child during this period.
>
> It is essential that all procedures and sensations which may be experienced by the child be described in advance. The possible sensations of warmth, tingling in the extremities, auditory changes, and changes in perceived body weight should be described to the child in a very positive manner. The use of good, positive descriptions will make the most of children's susceptibility to suggestion. Using language and concepts which the child can understand, such as comparing the experience to that of pilots and astronauts, simplifies the introduction.

Moreover, Barenie (1979) notes that during introductory administration, the child's reactions should be monitored. He/she should be questioned about his/her feelings, and a "continuing description of sensations he/she may become aware of should be related." Sorenson and Roth's (1973) suggestions on how to introduce nitrous oxide demonstrate appreciation of the role of psychological preparation for both adults and children. Their first three steps are as follows:

1. Seat the patient comfortably in the chair.

2. Check openings of inspiratory valve and tension of expiratory valve on nasal inhaler for suggested settings. Open tanks and check pressure gauges for adequate levels of gases.

3. Predict symptoms the individual will feel and tell him or her s/he will experience a pleasant sensation, a tingling sensation in toes, fingertips, on the tongue, and on the upper lip. Use a pleasant, controlled tone of voice.

Other experts, such as Langa (1968) and Allen (1979), maintain that the administration of nitrous oxide-oxygen mixture should be accompanied by supportive dentist behaviors and the patient told about its beneficial effects. It is not unreasonable to believe, therefore, that when nitrous oxide sedation is effective in reducing the distress of patients, it may be that the effect is the result of the non-pharmacologic management technique as well as that of the drug.

PLACEBOS. Another closely related and time-honored method for managing pain involves placebos. Placebo effect may be defined as one which is not due to specific pharmacological properties of a drug. The placebo effect is readily produced by suggestion in the context of the clinical and experimental situations. Placebo responsiveness has been well documented. Beecher (1972) has shown that 35 percent of patients obtain pain relief with placebos. The greater the anxiety, the greater is the relief from placebo medications. Evans (1974) reported the relative efficiency of placebos and drugs such as morphine, Darvon®, or aspirin as .54–.56. That is, a placebo is 56 percent as effective as morphine. The effectiveness of a placebo is directly proportional to the active analgesic agent with which it is being compared. A placebo is usually more effective in relieving severe pain. The properties of the placebo mimic the drug with which it is being compared. Effects of the placebo and the comparison drug usually interact and are additive. Higher placebo dosages are more effective than lower dosages. Injections are more effective than orally given placebos. Placebos are more effective under double-blind conditions, when neither the dentist nor patient know of their content. Placebos are also more effective when described to patients as powerful than when described as experimental. They are also more effective when given by a physician who is more likely to prescribe drugs.

At times we use suggestion and capitalize upon the placebo effect for anxiety and pain control. Drug-oriented patients concerned about previous anesthetic failure are provided with "special" anesthetics. Similarly, early in treatment, anxious patients who have occasionally taken tranquilizers do very well on 5 mg of diazepam taken upon arrival at the clinic, usually 30 minutes prior to being seated in the dental chair. However, placebos may not be very effective with patients with chronic anxiety and long-term use of tranquilizing drugs. Such patients may find placebos worsen their anxiety state (Riekels and Downing, 1967).

In summary, patient expectations influence the pain experience. How we prepare patients for our treatments will influence, to a great extent, what they feel. Suggestion, placebo, and hypnosis are useful in control of pain, which must be dealt with in almost every phase of dentistry. While pain itself can be controlled by drugs, anxiety and the fear of pain must be controlled psychologically.

CONCLUSION

The objective of this chapter is to provide a clinical link between fear, described in Chapters 1 and 2, and pain. We take this approach because pain is a common presenting complaint when we see fearful patients, and because most fearful persons will be anxious about being hurt by the dentist. Many patients will report being hurt previously in dental treatment.

We show here that pain is a broad clinical phenomenon and stress that it is much more than a one-to-one stimulation-reception phenomenon. Pain involves cognitive processes as well. Cultural background, personality, coping styles, and suggestibility are all factors that influence the pain response.

A second objective of this chapter is to discuss pain control. Effective pain control is important clinically because it allows the fearful patient to experience dental treatment in comfort. For many, several pain-free sessions will eliminate much of the fear response. In this chapter we discuss the use of local anesthetics and ancillary agents. Drug formulations, dosage, time until onset, duration and area of anesthesia are covered. Newer long acting anesthetics are included in the discussion.

Particular attention is directed to two types of common clinical problems—inadequate anesthesia and adverse effects. We find, on average, 13 percent of patients are treated by dentists without adequate anesthesia—anesthetic failure. Suggestions are made to prevent this problem clinically. Similarly untoward effects—palpitations, sweating, nausea, dizziness, and fainting—are relatively common. The chapter contains clinical information on allergic, toxic, and psychogenic reactions and how to identify and treat them psychologically and pharmacologically.

Finally, clinical suggestions are made about how to use ancillary pharmacologic agents such as diazepam and nitrous oxide as part of behavioral strategies. The role of the placebo is discussed.

Pain is a complex clinical problem, but the dental profession has available some very effective behavioral and pharmacologic tools for pain control. Used correctly, these modalities offer the fearful patient a potentially pain free experience which (we shall see in later chapters) is essential to recovery from the disability and discomfort of dental fear.

QUESTIONS AND EXERCISES

1. Consider the pain you might experience and your reaction to twisting your ankle while playing volleyball or basketball with a group of friends. How would you respond and what would you say? How might your reaction differ from that of a seven-year-old child in the same situation? What factors would affect how you responded? Consider your family, cultural background, your personality, and the situation in which you experienced the pain. Who do you know who would respond differently? How? Why?

2. How might you determine if your patients are sensitizers or monitors or repressors/blunters? Consider how persons who differ in these ways might require different approaches on your part to the introduction of local anesthesia.

3. List several steps described in this chapter that may enhance the effects of local anesthetic. Describe specifically how you would implement these steps.

4. Describe the circumstances under which ancillary agents such as nitrous oxide or diazepam might be useful clinically.

5. Describe how you would respond to a new patient who informs you that he or she is "allergic to Novocaine" and/or does not want epinephrine in the local anesthetic.

FOUR

Assessing the Problem: Understanding the Patient's Fears

GENERAL CONSIDERATIONS

In the preceding chapters, we discussed conceptual models to explain the processes underlying fear and pain. These models provide a framework for understanding clinical problems.

Now we will focus on the application of these concepts to assess dental fear. The first step is to conduct a thorough examination of the problem. This may occur in a variety of ways. For example, in order to determine the status of a particular tooth you may utilize an explorer, periodontal probe, X-rays, and pulp tester. The process of evaluating the psychological state of a patient is no different from the diagnostic process used for determining the health status of a tooth, only the tools differ.

Thus, in working with the fearful patient, the dental procedure does not change; you simply have an additional set of data: the patients' fears. With the very fearful patient, this may be the crucial factor determining the probability of success with a patient.

Anxiety is generally referred to by laymen as though it connotes a specific set of feelings and behaviors. Although such usage is common, it belies the complexity of the concept. It is critical to realize that the labels *anxiety* and *fear* are general concepts for a variety of feelings and behaviors. Recall anxiety is a response in anticipation of a dreaded event, while fear is the response in the presence of the stressor. Both problems are discussed in this and the following chapters. Some patients may have an overriding fear of pain, while others will report a fear of feeling totally helpless or claustrophobic. It is crucial to understand that the fears and anxieties of patients may differ from one another although they all have a common theme of dental fear. It is also important to realize, as discussed in Chapter 1, that signs of fear can be expressed by an individual in three different areas. These areas are: *the patient's behavior*—what we see the patient do—such as gripping the chair arms tightly; *the patient's physiological responses*—such as rapid breathing or profuse sweating; and *the patient's self-report*—what the patient says about his fear. When taken together, signs from these three areas indicate the presence of a constellation of emotions we label as fear. A patient's fear may be expressed in any one of these areas alone or in combination. A patient, for example, may report feeling terrified and yet appear calm and physiologically unaroused while in the chair.

We present here a useful diagnostic approach that groups patient fears into four types. To work successfully with the fearful patient, we use management techniques appropriate to the specific type of fear. A diagnosis is useful only if it leads to differing treatment strategies. Similarly, when confronted with a complex restorative problem, such as missing teeth, a skilled clinician will take into consideration a multitude of factors. Knowing there may be a number of possible solutions to the problem, the practitioner may weigh the patient's concern with esthetics, health care habits, financial resources, and gingival health prior to deciding on an appropriate treatment strategy to recommend. A somewhat less skilled clinician, however, may attempt to treat similar technical problems the same way each time based on a fixed ideal of "the way it was taught in school," or of a personal philosophy of "I do only first-class 'Cadillac' restorative work." Each of us has probably seen examples of technically excellent dental work where the plan was inappropriate for the particular patient. Just the same, in the treatment of a fearful patient there is no single approach that works equally well with every patient. The application of appropriate treatment strategies specific to both the patient and the problem will be discussed in detail in Chapters 5–9. Special strategies for children are in Chapter 10.

UNIVERSITY OF WASHINGTON DIAGNOSTIC CATEGORIES OF DENTAL FEAR

This classification system attempts to bring order to a complex area of behavior. The specific clinical strategies suggested in the later chapters are based on these diagnostic categories. Note that these categories are not psychiatric or psychological diagnostic classifications and are not intended as such. They were developed out of our work with patients and have proved clinically useful in treatment. Our purpose here is not to turn the dental reader into a psychologist but to provide an understanding of the differences between patients. We must also emphasize that people (and their fears) seldom come in neat packages. An individual may exhibit fears from more than one category.

We will now discuss four diagnostic categories of fear. It is useful to think of each category having as its root a specific kind of fear. However, as described in Chapter 2, lack of control over the dentist is a theme common to all types.

The first category is the *fear of specific stimuli*; it is based on the fear of being unable to tolerate discomfort associated with dental treatment. Second is *distrust* of the dental provider. Based on an inability to communicate, this category may include one or more of the following: a loss of self-esteem as a result of perceived belittlement; a feeling of helplessness and lack of control in the dental situation; or suspicion and doubt of what the dentist says and does. Third, there is the category we call *generalized anxiety*. Patients in this category find many different situations to be difficult and stressful. They worry and anticipate the worst. Such patients believe they cannot adequately control their own upsetting thoughts which are the cause of their fear. The final category is the *fear of a medically or emotionally overwhelming catastrophe*. It is based on a fear of having an uncontrollable bodily reaction to dental treatment, such as a heart attack, choking, or a panic attack.

We will now examine each category in more detail. Below are composite descriptions of patients representative of each of the four categories of fear. The descriptions are, so far as possible, in the patient's own words in order to present a clinical picture of how these patients appear in the dental office. The descriptions are organized into patient's dental history, presenting complaint, medical history, and social-psychological status. How to elicit relevant information in the assessment process is discussed following the descriptions.

Fear of Specific Stimuli

DENTAL HISTORY. "I had horrible experiences with drilling as a kid. My dentist never used Novacaine and held me down. I haven't gone regularly since my mother quit dragging me. I only go when I'm in so much pain that I finally can't take it any longer." "All my experiences have been very painful. I hardly ever get numb. . . ." "I don't mind the dentistry; I never have been able to stand the shots."

PRESENTING COMPLAINT. "I hate all of dentistry (nothing personal). I have a low pain tolerance. I don't mind anything except the pain." "The dentist would tell me it wouldn't hurt. . . . I have a difficult time getting numb. . . . I'd rather go a few weeks with a toothache than go through that pain." "I just hate those injections."

MEDICAL HISTORY. Within normal limits. Some patients report difficulties with specific medical procedures, such as injections and blood drawing.

SOCIAL/PSYCHOLOGICAL HISTORY. "I can't think of anything else I'm afraid of besides dentistry."

APPROPRIATE TREATMENT STRATEGIES. SEE CHAPTER 6.

Distrust of Dental Personnel

DENTAL HISTORY. "My dentist wasn't interested in me. He made fun of my fears. . . . He didn't let me ask questions . . . always in a hurry. He always said, 'Keep open, just a little longer.' A little longer to him was a lot longer to me." "The dentist would hide the needle and surprise me. . . . His hygienist would make me feel guilty about how I was caring for my teeth."

PRESENTING COMPLAINT. "I want to be treated as a person. . . . It's important to me that I am able to communicate." "He treated me just like another set of teeth." "My dentist would become impatient if I asked questions." "I guess I really have felt put down and now I am unable to trust dentists." "They always made me feel guilty about the way I cared for my teeth." "The dentist made fun of my fears and said I was being a baby."

MEDICAL HISTORY. Within normal limits. There may be distrust of medical personnel.

SOCIAL/PSYCHOLOGICAL HISTORY. May appear to be cynical or angry. Sensitive to being taken advantage of in a variety of life circumstances.

APPROPRIATE TREATMENT STRATEGIES. SEE CHAPTER 7.

Generalized Anxiety

DENTAL HISTORY. "I have to come in to get my teeth cleaned and x-rayed. But when they tell me about the work that needs to be done I never go back. . . . I've always hated going, but it's getting worse." "I make appointments and then don't show up or cancel at the last moment. . . . I'm a wreck for a week before my appointment."

PRESENTING COMPLAINT. "Everything about dentistry is awful . . . and I know I have a ton of work that needs to be done. I can't really bear to think about it; it's too upsetting." "I can't stop thinking about it." "I worry about it . . . all the time. I've always had problems with my teeth. It's a nightmare."

MEDICAL HISTORY. Patient will frequently have numerous chronic somatic complaints and conditions such as: headaches, bowel and digestive problems, allergies, swollen joints, asthma. There may be a long medical treatment history with many different physicians. Patient will often have been checked out for a variety of medical conditions, the results of which may have been mostly negative. They are the group of patients who are most likely to be taking various antianxiety drugs such as Valium® or Elavil®.

SOCIAL/PSYCHOLOGICAL HISTORY. "I'm a worrier. I get anxious about the future. . . . I tend to anticipate and ruminate over problems. . . . I'm high strung." "I don't handle stress very well. There are a lot of stressful things happening in my life. I cry easily. . . . I get depressed fairly often. . . . I'm afraid of other things besides dentistry (most commonly fear of heights, closed spaces, and flying). I find it hard to tell other people what I really want . . . when I have a problem I wind up sticking my head in the sand and hope it will go away."

APPROPRIATE TREATMENT STRATEGIES. SEE CHAPTER 8.

Fear of Catastrophe

DENTAL HISTORY. "I've had a lot of dental work done, but several years ago I began to have these terrible physical reactions to dental treatment which got worse and worse until I finally stopped going. Some of my attacks were so bad I had to leave in the middle of the appointment. . . . The dentist sent me home after I fainted in the chair and had me go see a physician!" "I get very panicky. . . . I know it was silly but I was afraid I couldn't breathe. I had to get out of there. . . . I was embarrassed. . . ."

PRESENTING COMPLAINT. "I think I'm allergic to the anesthetic. . . . I'm not afraid of dentistry; I'm afraid of having an attack." "I feel like I might gag or choke to death. I was okay until he put on the rubber dam."

MEDICAL HISTORY. Patient will frequently have a history of "attacks" in various situations and tendency to attribute physical causes to these. Common physical reactions include: rapid heart rate, hyperventilation, numbness and tingling of extremities, perceived difficulty in breathing, choking, gagging, gasping for air. He may have history of consulting a variety of medical specialists about the problem. Patient will often report allergic reactions to a wide variety of substances. He may have undiagnosed cardiac disease such as mitral valve prolapse.

SOCIAL/PSYCHOLOGICAL HISTORY. Patient's history will generally appear within normal limits except for this one area. Patient will frequently be able to talk quite rationally about the problem. The individual will frequently restrict himself from certain types of activities that he feels might set off such attacks.

APPROPRIATE TREATMENT STRATEGIES. SEE CHAPTER 9.

DISTINGUISHING CHARACTERISTICS OF THE FOUR CATEGORIES

The above descriptions were presented *primarily* by patients describing themselves. Prior to discussing how to make a diagnosis, we will summarize the distinguishing characteristics of each category, especially as they relate to the fear of loss of control. In Figure 4-1 is a checklist which is filled out in the DFRC following the assessment interview. It presents in outline the principal fears associated with each category.

Fear Of Specific Stimuli

Pain and the fear of feeling pain are usually mentioned first when patients are asked why they fear dental care. This is the "expected" answer and is almost always a *contributing* factor. However, it is important to assess if pain is the *predominant* fear. When it *is* of primary concern, patients are likely to say such things as: "It is the pain. What else is there?" They are emphatic that pain is what they fear. These patients can usually trace the origin of their fears to specific experiences: "When I was 14 years old, the dentist pulled my tooth without me being numb. . . ." The fear of pain is focused around a very specific agent such as the needle or drilling.

   CONTROL. Patients with this fear as their principal concern are worried the pain will be too intense to bear. They fear they will have no way to prevent the experience from being aversive.

Distrust of Dental Personnel

These patients are hypersensitive to the behavior of dental personnel. They frequently report that "their former dentist didn't care about them,"

DIAGNOSIS CHECKLIST

Check major type(s) and subcategories as appropriate:

I. Fear of Specific Stimulus

_____ pain: mistakes, incompetence of dentist

_____ pain: (simple) fear of physical sensation

     _____ drilling   _____ vibration

     _____ noise   _____ needle

     _____ cleaning   _____ impressions

. . . fear of inability to
       tolerate sensation

Comment: _____

II. Distrust of Dental Personnel

_____ belittlement of fears

_____ belittlement of oral care habits/health

_____ dentist won't respond to concerns even if expressed or take
     seriously.

_____ fear of inability to stop/control dentist (victim)

_____ not treated as individual / as person

_____ dentist takes fears personally / responds with anger, frus-
     tration

. . health professional's
       verbalizations

. . . loss of self-esteem

. . . loss of control

Comment: _____

112

III. Generalized Anxiety
_____ multiple fears/phobias: _____ . . . "everything"
_____ . . . one's thoughts & feelings
_____ multiple sources of perceived stress _____ . . . feelings of inadequacy

_____ inadequate coping skills (describes self as extremely nervous type)
_____ anticipatory worrying/physical symptoms of
_____ fear of enormity of problem, "bad news"
_____ other psychological problems: hypochondriasis, depression
Comment: _____

IV. Fear of Catastrophe _____ . . . one's own bodily reactions
_____ death, hyperallergic reaction, gagging, choking, etc.
_____ being overwhelmed, _having_ panic attack (fear of fear)
_____ fear of embarrassing self, appearing silly
Comment: _____

FIGURE 4-1. Dental Fears Research Clinic Checklist.

113

the dental hygienist "acted like she wished I could drop my teeth off at the door in the morning," or the receptionist "tried to pull a fast one." They often mention feeling guilty, or being put down for their home oral care: "I *know* my teeth are terrible, I don't need anyone to make me feel worse," or "The dentist took my fears personally and got angry because I was afraid."

These patients may report experiences where the dentist told them, "Stop acting like a baby," or to "grow up." They may feel the dentist is trying to fool them by hiding the syringe and sneaking it in. These patients are concerned with loss of self-esteem and an inability to interact meaningfully with the health professional. They have a *low* level of trust and are cynical of reassurances about how "everything will be O.K."

CONTROL. Patients in this cateogry feel dental personnel are authoritarian and will do whatever they wish, no matter what the patient says or does. They describe themselves as feeling like a victim, at the whim or mercy of the dentist. This attitude is frequently a result of repeated negative childhood experiences with a particular individual.

Generalized Anxiety

These patients' fears appear to be more general. Many situations are perceived as stressful. Your first impression is that they don't cope with stress very well.

Dental fear may be the predominant one but is usually one of several fears. The patient is likely to describe an entire experience as scary, but is unable to describe exactly what about it is so frightening. He focuses on his worry and anticipation rather than what to do about the problem. Such patients are likely to report being worried about an appointment several days prior to coming in. They frequently mention not sleeping well the night before the visit. Patients in this group are likely to report canceling previous dental appointments. It is also common for them to report other situations in which they are fearful. The most common are flying, heights, and closed spaces.

HERMAN®

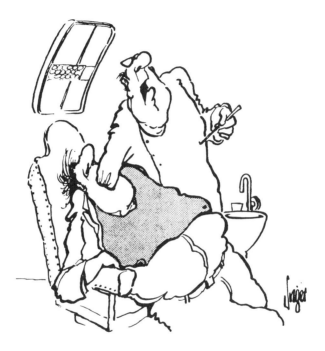

"Hold still! I dropped my little mirror."

CONTROL. Patients with this category feel their *thoughts* are not controllable. They may say things like, "My thoughts run away on their own." "I can't stop thinking/worrying about it." They see events and situations as beyond their personal control because of their own inadequacies. They know that other people can deal with the dental situation; it is their own abilities they doubt. Thus, the fear of dentistry is not usually a result of a specific trauma. Rather, it is more generally poor coping abilities causing difficulty in several areas of the individual's life.

Fear of Catastrophe

Patients whose fears fall within this category report being afraid of experiencing a life-threatening medical emergency during dental treatment. In extreme cases they fear dying in the chair from a heart attack or cerebral aneurysm. They are attuned to bodily sensations: heart palpitations, numbness of extremities, profuse sweating, or chills. Patients who report that they are allergic to the anesthetic and that it causes their heart to beat uncontrollably, or that it causes them difficulty in breathing, also fall within this category. Finally, there are some patients who believe that the dentist will make a horrible mistake resulting in a medical emergency.

CONTROL. Almost without exception, these patients feel their bodily responses are beyond volitional control. They frequently have a history of "attacks," or "reactions" and are afraid their body will "run amuck." They fear fainting, not being able to breathe, or choking to death. Patients who attribute their reactions to a physical stimulus or physiological reaction will frequently state they are *not* afraid of dentistry, only their involuntary bodily response. Other patients, however, primarily fear they will lose control emotionally and act irrationally by fleeing, crying, or screaming, or otherwise acting childishly and embarrass themselves. Over time, both kinds of panic patients learn to identify what triggers the incidents but believe that once "started down the path" it is uncontrollable until it has run its course. To borrow a phrase, these patients have a *fear of fear*. In order to avoid such attacks, these individuals avoid any situation that might trigger an episode.

Now that we have described major diagnostic categories, we turn to the process of determining in which category an individual patient best fits. There are three steps in the assessment process. First is the recognition of the basic signs of anxiety. Second is the psychological examination and diagnosis. Third is choosing the appropriate treatment strategies specific to fear.

THE ASSESSEMENT PROCESS IN THE OFFICE

General Considerations

There are three points at which you can identify the fearful patient. The patient may be identified as fearful *after* treatment has begun. Alternatively, determination may be made *during* the initial appointment. Finally, it is possible to identify patients as fearful *prior* to their first visit. Obviously, the *earlier* you are able to determine that the patient is fearful, the greater the probability of success in working with that patient. Consequently, we will first examine how you can identify and then work with the new fearful patient.

There are three primary sources of information for making an assessment. They are, as mentioned previously, *self-report* (what the patient tells you), *behavioral signs*, and *physiological indicators*. Signs in any one or combination of these systems may indicate the presence of fear. Note that any one sign, taken by itself, tells us little without other information. Confounding the problem of identifying anxiety is that responses in these three areas do not always occur simultaneously (Rachman and Hodgson, 1974a,b). That is, a person might deny or not admit that he or she is particularly fearful, yet show significant physiological changes when seated in the operatory. This is particularly true when fear levels are moderate. Similarly, one might come yearly for an examination, behave like a model patient, yet report being terrified. To complicate things further, different patients respond with different physiological signs when upset. For example, one patient might break out in sweat but show relatively little change in heart rate, while another might have quite the opposite pattern. This lack of strict correspondence among and within the various systems indicative of fear can lead to erroneous assumptions concerning the actual psychological state of the patient. Overall, though sometimes contrary to our

117

sense and instruments, we believe that it is best to trust the self-report of the patient.

Recognizing the Basic Signs of Anxiety

SELF REPORT. The patient serves as a primary source of information. However, such information cannot always be taken at face value. The conditions under which such reports are obtained can influence the content and validity of the information. If the patient is afraid of appearing silly or feels uncomfortable talking with you, he or she may say nothing about, or minimize, his or her fears.

Self-reports concerning fear of dentistry can be obtained through an intake interview, questionnaires, or phone follow-ups. We will first examine the intake interview.

The best time to identify the fearful patient is prior to a visit during the initial telephone contact. This is not difficult. By adding a few questions to the information the receptionist normally obtains prior to the first appointment, the majority of fearful patients can be identified. Below are listed questions that might be included in the initial telephone intake.

1. How long has it been since your last dental visit?

2. What kind of treatment did you have? How was it? How did it feel?

3. Do you have any concerns about receiving dental treatment that would be helpful for us to know?

Question 1: How long has it been since your last dental visit? That is, why did the patient decide to make an appointment at this time—rather than six months ago or six months in the future? The patient is encouraged to describe his or her most recent appointment and feelings about it. Patients often report they have come in because "A filling fell out a few months ago," "I've been having a dull ache for a week," or "I've been putting it off for years and I know I have lots of problems, so I finally forced myself to come." "I came because my spouse asked me to."

118

Fearful patients often wait until they think something is wrong. If the patient has recently been to another dentist he or she may have been "dissatisfied" or had a traumatic experience with that dentist.

Question 2: *What kind of treatment did you have? How was it? How did you feel?* It is important to remember that you are seeking the patient's perception of the experience, how he or she remembers it. You may know (or think you do) that the report is exaggerated or could not be accurate. This is unimportant at this point. Your task is not to try and correct their misunderstandings or doubt the experience. Instead, it is to understand how the patient perceives the experience. Another key question is "How did you hear of us?" It is important for any practice to know how patients find you; but in the case of a fearful patient, it may let you know they called specifically because of your reputation for working with fearful patients. Alternatively, you may have your receptionist make some kind of statement to each person seeking an appointment such as: "I don't know if you are aware of this, but our dentist has a special interest in working with people who are apprehensive of dental treatment. How have you felt about going to the dentist?"

For those offices which routinely provide a packet of materials for the first-time patient to complete prior to the first visit, we recommend the use of the Corah Dental Anxiety Scale. One of the most widely used and researched, it is short and easy to complete. As you can see in Figure 4-2, its primary focus is on the anticipation of dental treatment. The research indicates that it is highly correlated with observed and reported dental anxiety (Corah et al. 1978).

Many people, of course, even though not particularly fearful, report that they do not enjoy going to the dentist. Screening questions help identify those individuals who find dentistry truly aversive and are willing to admit it. Identifying such patients prior to their first appointment allows you to structure their dental experience differently from the regular patient.

Prior to examining the use of self-report techniques in the initial appointment and during treatment, we will first review the behavioral and

1. If you had to go to the dentist tomorrow, how would you feel about it?
   a. I would look forward to it as a reasonably enjoyable experience.
   b. I wouldn't care one way or the other.
   c. I would be a little uneasy about it.
   d. I would be afraid that it would be unpleasant and painful.
   e. I would be very frightened of what the dentist might do.

2. When you are waiting in the dentist's office for your turn in the chair, how do you feel?
   a. Relaxed.
   b. A little uneasy.
   c. Tense.
   d. Anxious.
   e. So anxious that I sometimes break out in a sweat or almost feel physically sick.

3. When you are in the dentist's chair waiting while he gets his drill ready to begin working on your teeth, how do you feel? (Same alternatives as number 2.)

4. You are in the dentist's chair to have your teeth cleaned. While you are waiting and the dentist is getting out the instruments which he will use to scrape your teeth around the gums, how do you feel? (Same alternatives as number 2.)

Points were assigned for the subject's choices, with one point for an (a) choice to 5 points for an (e) choice.

From Corah, N.L.; Assessment of a dental anxiety scale, *Journal of Dental Research*, 48:496, July–August 1969. Reprinted with permission.

FIGURE 4-2. *Corah Dental Anxiety Scale.*

physiological signs of anxiety, signs which can be observed when the patient first comes to your office.

BEHAVIORAL SIGNS. The patient's behavior in the waiting room can provide an early indication of whether or not he or she is anxious.

However, as in the case with other types of information, waiting room behavior itself can only be considered as a possible sign of anxiety. Nonetheless, there are data suggesting that fearful patients display more movement in the waiting room than do non-fearful patients (Barash, 1974; Kleinknecht and Bernstein, 1978). In particular, fearful patients frequently display more arm and hand movements than non-fearful patients rapidly thumbing through magazines and fidgeting with their hands or other objects.

Because the person in the most advantageous position to observe patients in the waiting room is the receptionist, he or she could make a note to cue the other staff members to explore the issue further before beginning the dental examination or treatment. Also, if from the earlier phone interview it was determined that the patient had not been to a dentist for several years, or had problems with previous dentists, behavioral observation could help confirm dental fear.

Figure 4-3 is a checklist of behavioral signs of anxiety that might be observed in the waiting room by the receptionist.

If the receptionist is included in the fear assessment team, it may be

---

BEHAVIOR CHECKLIST

Pt. Name   _____   fidgeting with hands or objects

_____   _____   sitting on edge of chair leaning forward

     _____   rapidly thumbing through magazines

Date   _____   pacing

_____   _____   frequent changes in sitting position

     _____   startled reactions to ordinary office noises

     _____   rapid head movement

     _____   repetitious hand/leg and foot movement

     _____   other

FIGURE 4-3. Checklist To Be Used By Receptionist.

helpful to use a form, such as the one above, to be given to the first clinician scheduled to see the patient. Once again, however, we caution against premature judgments based only on waiting room behavior. Patients may be active and anxious for reasons other than impending dentistry. For example, they might have experienced a near auto accident on their way to the office or might be concerned about being late to another appointment. Moreover, some displays of anger are very similar to anxious behavior and may or may not be related to dental fear.

Interestingly, in Chapter 1 we reported a study showing that specific behaviors asssociated with fear in the operatory take essentially the opposite pattern from what occurred in the waiting room. That is, high fear patients moved less, talked to the dentist or assistant less, and held their hands clasped more than low fear patients. These patients may appear tense or rigid. Further, the behaviors that most clearly differentiate high from low fear patients occur prior to actual treatment when the patient is alone in the operatory or when either the dentist or the assistant is present but not yet involved in treatment.

Observation of patient behavior in the operatory provides the opportunity to further test out a hypothesis and to discuss observations with the patient either at that time, or if more privacy and detailed discussion appear warranted, during a more extensive interview.

PHYSIOLOGICAL SIGNS. Activiation of the autonomic nervous system (ANS) under stress provides another constellation of fear indicators. Under ideal conditions, changes in organ systems innervated by the ANS can be precisely monitored with a polygraph. Unfortunately, such instrumentation is both too cumbersome and expensive for routine use in a dental office. However, signs of ANS activation are readily observable.

There are three physiological indicators that can readily be observed in the office. One of the most clearly observable signs is excessive perspiration. Those areas particularly sensitive to "arousal sweating" (Kuno, 1956) include the palms of the hands, underarms, forehead, and upper portions of the lip. The latter two are observable, the former easily assessed by a handshake.

The second set of signs are the cardiovascular responses. They include pulse rate and blood pressure. For patients whose fears focus around catastrophic physical reactions we frequently utilize a portable heart rate monitor to provide them feedback. Pulsation in the carotid and temporal arteries can also be observed from the dentist's typical working position. Observation of arterial pulsation has the advantage of being unobtrusive and can be done periodically to assess changes throughout an appointment.

Finally, observation of the depth and rate of respiration can provide yet another index of anxiety. Rapid, shallow breathing suggests increased arousal. Similarly, situations in which the patient *holds* his breath is a common sign of fear. This is most likely to occur during a procedure in which the patient fears he may be hurt, i.e., in the injection or during extraction. These observations may be most effectively made by the assistant while the dentist is involved in the treatment procedures.

A FEAR ASSESSMENT INTERVIEW

Objectives of a Fear Assessment Interview

1. To visibly demonstrate to the patient that you are concerned with finding out who he or she is, and what his or her concerns are.

2. To begin establishing a relationship of trust based upon two-way communication.

3. To let the patient know that his or her worries/concerns are taken seriously and are considered "normal."

4. To obain the patient's point of view or perspective on the nature and extent of the problem.

5. To obtain sufficient information to arrive at an assessment or diagnosis of the nature and type of fear exhibited by the patient.

6. To obtain a sense of the patient's dental I.Q.—his or her understanding of their current problems and knowledge of dental disease and prevention.

7. To gain an understanding of how the patient copes with stressful situations.

General Considerations

In many dental practices it is customary to schedule non-emergency patients automatically for a hygienist appointment and radiographs prior to the initial examination by the dentist. For the "regular" dental patient or "goers but haters" this may prove satisfactory. However, for the fearful patient this approach will frequently cause problems. A patient who has a fear of bad news, for example, may work himself into such an anxious state by the time you are ready to make a case presentation that he will be unable to attend to what is actually said. A distrustful but non-assertive individual may feel he or she is getting the runaround by being seen only by auxiliary personnel.

Although it may appear at first glance to be a somewhat unusual suggestion, our experience has led us to the conclusion that those patients who you strongly feel may be fearful should be interviewed prior to *any* treatment, including an examination. The initial relationship established will, more than any other factor, determine if the patient will enter and ultimately remain in your practice. Preferably, this interview is held outside the operatory in a consultation room. In those offices where this is not possible, we recommend that the patient be allowed to sit upright in the chair and that an atmosphere of privacy, so far as possible, be established. The interview could be done by the hygienist or dentist. Who does the interview is less important than how it is conducted.

Remember, many patients are somewhat reluctant to admit to others that they are fearful. They have frequently received the message from friends or other dentists that they should stop being childish and "learn how to control themselves." Consequently, the more private the interview setting, the more comfortable and open your prospective patient is likely to be.

CAVEAT. Whenever you reach a point, no matter what you are doing, that you suspect a patient is fearful, it is important to quickly but gently check out your observations. You may simply report what you see. "You seem to be grasping the chair very tightly," or, "You seem to be holding your breath when I work." Alternatively, inquire directly about

124

how the patient is feeling, "Are you feeling a little nervous about the appointment today?" If a patient responds in a way to confirm your observations, it is time to lay down your dental instruments, sit the patient up, and begin talking! It doesn't matter if you are scheduled to do a MO on #28. Your purpose changes from getting a dental procedure completed to ensuring that the patient has a non-traumatic experience.

Introducing the Interview

What can you say to the patient about your desire to interview him or her about "feelings about the dentist"? Imagine the following conversation:

Dentist: John, from some of the things you have said, it seems like you are a little anxious about having dental work done.

John: Well, yes, but then I guess everybody is a little nervous about it.

Dentist: True, but some people get more anxious than others, and before I devise a treatment plan or begin work, I would like to take a few minutes to ask you a few questions which help me know how to make your experience here as comfortable as I can. Is that OK with you?

John: Sure, why not?

Dentist: OK, good. My purpose is first to try to figure out what I can do to make treatment as easy and comfortable for you as possible. Secondly, I want to see if I can figure out what you might do for yourself to successfully cope with what many patients find to be a stressful situation.

It is also critical somewhere prior to or near the beginning of the interview to convey to the patient that you take their worries and concerns seriously. That is, you recognize they are legitimate, real, and "normal." Now it may be that some of you may be feeling that the patients fears are *exaggerated*. After all, operative dentistry is familiar, and you know how safe, painless, and easy it can be. However, "objective facts," or what *you* know, have little influence on another person's fears. To make this clear, we often use the analogy of flying. For example we might say, "I am sure you have heard about or know someone who is terrified of flying. And even though they know the most dangerous part about air travel is driving to the airport, they will not fly. Well, it is reasonable to be somewhat afraid of flying. It *can* be dangerous and there is little you could do if things went wrong. Thus, even though the chance of something going wrong is very low, it is natural to feel some apprehension about it. Dentistry is similar. It is a little scary to be on your back, with people leaning over you. Some things about dentistry are uncomfortable." The key point is to have the patient understand that you accept in a non-judgmental way that he is afraid and that you can work with him to help him overcome it.

Figure 4-4 lists a series of questions useful in an initial assessment interview. Obviously, not every question is asked of every new patient. However, the questions provide a basis for obtaining the information necessary to make an accurate assessment of the patient. We will discuss each question in turn, looking at typical responses and how to begin to differentiate between different types of fear.

Question 1.   Why did you make an appointment at this time? Do you need dental treatment now?

Question 2.   a. When was your last dental visit? What did you have done? How did you feel?
b. Describe your last restorative appointment (date work performed, etc.).

You will recognize questions 1 and 2 as those we recommended your receptionist ask as part of the initial telephone intake. Even if they have been asked of the patient previously, the questions provide a good starting point, as well as allow you to hear in the patient's own words why he or she made an appointment to come to the dentist at this time. By asking, "Why now instead of six months ago, or six months from now," you have an opportunity to understand the importance patients place on dental care and their feelings about it. Fearful patients generally wait until something

1. Why did you make an appointment at this time? Do you need dental treatment now?

2. a. When was your last dental visit? What did you have done? How did you feel?

   b. Describe your last restorative appointment (date work performed, etc.).

3. In general, what are the most difficult/fearful things about dentistry?

4. What kinds of things can the dentist say or do that make things worse?

5. What kinds of things can the dentist say or do that make receiving care easier?

6. What kinds of things, besides dentistry, are you afraid of?

7. How do you feel the night/morning before you are scheduled to come in for an appointment?

8. Are you more likely to delay making an appointment because of your feelings about dentistry? Or to cancel it after it is made?

9. Have you ever seriously considered having all your teeth pulled and getting dentures? Explain.

10. Are you interested in improving the appearance of your teeth? Explain.

11. Do you feel the appearance of your teeth limits your *activities* in any way? Explain.

12. In the last two years, has the condition of your teeth affected your health in such a way as to limit or cause you to cancel social activities or miss work? If yes, how much?

13. Are your friends or family aware of your fears? If so, what kinds of things have they said?

14. Do you feel that the condition of your teeth affects, in any way, your *relationships* with family or friends? Explain.

FIGURE 4-4. *Structured Interview.*

has gone wrong before they make an appointment. The average patient at the Dental Fears Research Clinic has not seen a dentist in about six years.

These questions allow you to explore a factor that frequently appears to be the primary concern and the basis of many patients' fears. It is the "fear of bad news." Have you ever had a series of headaches and thought "brain tumor"; persistent abdominal troubles and feared intestinal cancer; and yet found yourself reluctant to have a thorough examination? The fear of "finding out that it's really serious," and "they all have to be pulled," or that the sensitivity means "my teeth are full of cavities" contributes to the avoidance of care. Individuals who express a fear of the magnitude of the problem, and a desire to avoid knowing, typify responses given by persons falling within the generalized anxiety category.

Question 3.   In general, what are the most fearful things about dentistry?

With some very obvious exceptions, most patients will first mention the fear of pain. It is the expected response, and it is tempting to accept these initial statements at face value. It seems logical that pain would be the most fearful aspect of receiving dental care. However, with some skillful interviewing, you will find that for many patients this is only one of several issues. Thus, the task is to determine if fear of pain is primary, or only a contributing factor. As mentioned previously, Bernstein, Kleinknecht, and Alexander (1979) found that over 50 percent of one sample of fearful patients cited "dentists' personal behavior and professional characteristics" as contributing to their fear of dentistry. Follow up questions such as: "Besides the pain, is there anything else about the dental experience which is frightening or bothersome to you?" will often encourage the patient to explore his or her feelings.

Fear of specific stimuli patients, those who are in fact primarily afraid of pain, tend to give this message very clearly. They are likely to say something like, "I just can't stand pain. I have low pain tolerance in my mouth," or "If it just didn't hurt." These individuals are usually able to graphically relate past traumatic dental experiences.

Those patients afraid of a catastrophe have fears revolving around physiological sensations. They will report that they are afraid of "choking, having my heart burst, fainting, or having an allergic anesthetic reaction."

Patients who have difficulty in coping with many different kinds of events are less likely to give specific responses to the question. They may respond with statements like, "It wasn't that bad to tell you the truth, but I just couldn't make myself go again." "I don't know exactly why I hate it, I just do."

Patients who are distrustful and feel at the mercy of the dentist tend to say things such as, "I'm afraid of being helpless and trapped." "I hate to be made to feel guilty about my teeth." "My dentist would tell me it didn't hurt and it did!"

Frequently the issue of pain tolerance arises. Patients may mention that they have a high pain tolerance, except for in the mouth, or that their pain tolerance has been decreasing over the past few years. Or they may say they have a low pain tolerance. As explained in Chapter 3, the issue of pain tolerance is an area of intense debate and the subject of much research. What is known, however, is that pain tolerance is readily modified under varying conditions. For example, in the 1950's childbirth was considered too painful to tolerate without various nerve blocks and pain medications. Today, many women choose natural childbirth. The intervening factor? The mind set of the mother as influenced by childbirth training and practice. We will discuss in detail the importance of perception in pain tolerance in Chapter 6.

Question 4. *What kinds of things could I do or say to make it easier for you during the appointment?*

This question explores what it is about the health professional that the patient finds important. Fear of specific stimuli patients will emphatically state, "Don't hurt me!" Distrustful individuals, if they trust you enough to respond, will talk about what they did not like about previous dental personnel and what they want you to do differently. Often their ideas are realistic or attainable. Typical responses include: "Take time to explain," "Tell me the truth," "Give me alternatives to choose from," "Let me rest," "Treat me like a person." Individuals afraid of a medical emergency will ask you in some way to prevent their catastrophe by some technical solution such as using a different drug or different procedure. Generally anxious persons will have little to recommend. They may say, "I don't know," or "Is there some drug you could use to knock me out so I don't have to know what you do?"

Question 5. What kinds of things have dental personnel done or said to make appointments more difficult?

For some patients, the answers to this question will have been supplied in Question 3. However, for others the question can result in additional information. Distrustful individuals are most likely to respond to this question with specific, clear answers. Typical responses: "He acted like a robot," "Put me down," "Told me it didn't hurt and it did," "Made fun of my teeth," "He got made because I wasn't taking care of them, "Didn't listen," "Wouldn't stop," "Held me down," "Got angry when I cried." From this question you should obtain a list of what the patient is especially sensitive to and what not to do! Individuals within the other categories will often have little or nothing to say in response to this question beyond what was said in response to Question 3.

Question 6. What other kinds of things besides dentistry are you afraid of?

This question allows you to move beyond the specifics of dentistry. We find that it is important to mention specifically the most common fears: flying, heights, closed spaces, elevators, and crowds to bring to mind other areas of concern. Your purpose is to determine the range of the patient's fears. Fear of specific stimuli patients are very rarely seriously afraid of anything besides dentistry. What do we mean by "seriously afraid"? Many of us find certain situations uncomfortable. Fears which we would categorize as serious are those which are of sufficient strength as to limit the individual's activities in some way. If the patient can think of no other situation that he particularly fears, it is a reliable sign that his fears are dental-specific. Such individuals are among the easiest of all patients to treat once you can pinpoint the specific cause of the fears.

However, you will find that many patients are fearful of numerous situations and events. Individuals with multiple fears generally fall primarily within the Generalized Anxiety or Catastrophe categories. These

130

groups can be differentiated by understanding what the patient is afraid of across situations. Individuals afraid of catastrophe will mention a fear of having the same general physiological response that they have experienced in other situations. Individuals with general anxiety will focus on their inability to cope with difficult stressful situations.

When a patient "admits" to other fears, it is important to explore how they affect the person; how he or she copes with it. You might ask an exploratory queston such as: "When you find yourself in a stressful situation, how do you deal with it?" Generally anxious individuals respond by saying things like, "I try to ignore it." "I stick my head in the sand." "I do everything I can to avoid it." "I put it off as long as I can." The theme of their responses is that they do not cope very well. Occasionally, you may find a patient who once had a fear of flying, of heights, or of cuts, and has overcome it. This provides an opportunity for you to inquire about how he or she got over it. Besides being able to reinforce the idea that he or she can overcome their dental fear as well, you may gain some concrete ideas of how to approach the problem of dental fear. Finally, many patients have gone through or participated in any number of "difficult or challenging" experiences such as: natural childbirth, Toastmasters, self-defense courses, or mountain climbing. These require "coping skills" that can be brought to bear upon their fears of dentistry. When a patient reports specific fears besides dentistry, it indicates a more complex situation. At this point it is important to explore underlying commonalities. The most common theme that appears throughout the majority of patients is a fear of loss of control and a feeling of helplessness. When asked what it is they find so difficult about those situations they may say things like, "I guess I hate the feeling of being trapped," or "When problems start getting too big, I just stop thinking about them." Because of the central importance of the control issue we will discuss it later in this chapter when we look at paper and pencil assessment tools.

Question 7.   *How do you feel the night/morning before you are scheduled to come in for an appointment?*

and

Question 8.   Are you likely to delay making an appointment because of your feelings about dentistry or to cancel it after it is made?.

The two questions above help you explore the patient's thought experiences prior to the appointment. They can provide valuable clues on how the patient psyches himself or herself up for a bad experience in your office. It is typical of many individuals with generalized anxiety to report that they don't sleep, get nervous, restless, and have other physical symptoms prior to an appointment. They find themselves anticipating and worrying about what *might* happen. Because this patient finds it easy to avoid dental care, it is important to find out if your patient delays making appointments but is good about showing up, or if they are likely to fail to appear or cancel once an appointment is made. People know what their patterns are and will tell you if asked. Obviously, a person who cancels must be treated differently from the simple avoider, where the principal management technique is making sure the patient does not walk out of the office without another appointment. Other individuals, especially those who fear specific stimuli or are distrustful, are more likely to report that "I don't worry about the dental appointment until just before I get here."

Question 9.   Have you ever seriously considered having all your teeth pulled and getting dentures? Explain.

Question 10.   Are you interested in improving the appearance of your teeth? Explain.

Question 11.   Do you feel the appearance of your teeth limits your activities in any way? Explain.

Question 12.   In the last two years, has the condition of your teeth affected your health in such a way as to limit or cause you to cancel social activities or miss work? If yes, how much?

Question 13.   Are your friends or family aware of your fears? If so, what kinds of things have they said?

Question 14. *Do you feel that the condition of your teeth affects, in any way, your relationships with family or friends? Explain.*

The final area to be explored in the interview is what can be termed the patient's perceived cost of illness. They are designed to help you gain a better understanding of the patient's dental I.Q. and the importance that he or she places on his or her teeth. Many of our patients state that they have thought about having their teeth pulled. Others are terrified that their teeth will *have* to be pulled. Esthetics, of course, are very personal and a major factor in the kind of recommendations made. The "social cost" of fear to the patient is a factor that may frequently act as a motivating factor. Loss of function is tolerated as are the inevitable changes in diet. Many patients, however, are acutely aware of their "bad smiles" and feel self-conscious to the point of limiting social contact, especially with new people. Lowering of self-esteem is not infrequent. Self-consciousness in dining, bad breath, and the inability to smile are often seen as barriers to successful careers and relationships. These kinds of concerns do not appear related to any particular type of dental fear. The information obtained, however, does allow you to gain an understanding of what is important to the patient. For example, we may begin working on the anterior teeth, rather than other "more urgent" problems in order to give the patient a "high reward" during those first "high fear" appointments. The importance of modifying the treatment plan to suit the individual will be discussed in more detail in Chapter 5.

Concluding the Interview

The clinician's role to this point has been to listen—to gain an understanding of the patient's perspective. As the interview nears a conclusion, it becomes important to tie things together and explain in general terms how you work with fearful patients. It is helpful to summarize the conceptual framework you presented prior to the interview. For example, "We work with a patient in two ways. First, we attempt to figure out what we can do to make it easier for you to accept treatment. Scheduling, signal mechanisms, preset rest periods, lots of explanations, etc., are examples of 'modifying the treatment or the dentist.' Secondly, we try to ascertain what it is you can do for yourself to make it easier for you to get through the appointment. That is, how can we help strengthen your coping skills?"

It is also critical to set realistic expectations and to define what we mean by success. For example, we might say something like this: "The goal is *not* to have you feel no fear; that is, not to become fearless. We feel that a certain degree of wariness or alertness is adaptive and normal. It is natural to be a little apprehensive upon take-off as an airline passenger. Our goal is simply to reduce your fear to a more comfortable or more tolerable level to where you can accept treatment and seek it out on a preventive basis in the future. This we feel is a far more attainable and realistic goal."

Lastly, we explain the mechanics of how the practice operates, and present the diagnostic paper and pencil measures, which are our next topic of discussion.

PAPER AND PENCIL ASSESSMENT TOOLS

Following the conclusion of the interview at the Dental Fears Research Clinic, the patients are asked to complete a series of questionnaires to obtain specific information regarding patients' perceptions. We administer these following the initial interview rather than prior to it. We feel that if you have made the patient comfortable, you are more likely to get honest responses to questions about what are often perceived as embarrassing topics. The information that can be obtained from paper and pencil measures may also be acquired in a skillfully conducted interview. Why then use these measures? Partly because it is more efficient; but, more importantly, the responses provide a basis of comparison *between* patients, allowing you to assess the degree or severity of the patients' worries and fears and can be given later to determine patient progress in overcoming fear. Some of these surveys will now be discussed.

THE DENTAL FEAR SURVEY

The Dental Fear Survey (DFS) has been the subject of considerable research. It was the instrument used to provide much of the data on the prevalence of dental fear and on the specific aspect of dentistry that most people fear; it was presented in Chapter 1. The DFS is shown in Figure 4-5.

As you can see, the DFS surveys three areas pertaining to dental fear. The first two questions assess patients' reported avoidance of dentistry because of fear. Recall from Chapter 1 that 44 percent of a large sample reported having put off making an appointment due to fear and 14 percent reported having canceled one because of fear. Responses to these questions should provide you with some good indication of the patient's fear and avoidance behavior.

One area of the DFS (questions 3 to 7) allows patients to report the degree of felt arousal while undergoing dental treatment. As stated previously, individuals afraid of catastrophe are particularly attuned to their physiological states and will tend to mark the high end of these reaction scales. Consequently, this section should be particularly diagnostic for such patients. Also, some patients may also indicate marked physical activation while others may show such arousal physically but not be aware of it themselves. Consequently, just because a patient reports being tense or not tense, we cannot automatically assume that he is reporting accurately. For example, we recently saw a patient, diagnosed as a catastrophe type, whose heart rate increased from 80 to 120 beats per minute simply at the mention that we were going to give an injection. Even with this 50 percent increase the patient was unaware of the change. It was only after her heart rate reached 140 bpm that she reported feeling anxious! Patients who fear specific stimuli or who are distrustful may or may not report undue physiological responding.

The third section of the DFS (questions 8 to 19) allows the patient to indicate how much fear each of several dental situations and procedures causes for them. This information of course would be useful for the clinician to know before starting treatment and can provide a rational starting point to begin treatment of the dental fear.

The final question (#20) is a general summary question where the patient can indicate, overall, how much fear he or she experiences from dentistry. Responses to this question are highly correlated to the sum of the responses from the previous 19 items and can serve as a good overall indicator of the general state of the patient's fear.

Name_____

Date_____

The items in this questionnaire refer to various situations, feelings, and reactions related to dental work. Please rate your feeling or reaction on these items by *circling the number* (1, 2, 3, 4, or 5) of the category which most closely corresponds to your reaction.

1. Has fear of dental work ever caused you to put off making an appointment?

1	2	3	4	5
never	once or twice	a few times	often	nearly every time

2. Has fear of dental work ever caused you to cancel or not appear for an appointment?

1	2	3	4	5
never	once or twice	a few times	often	nearly every time

When having dental work done:

3. My muscles become tense

1	2	3	4	5
not at all	a little	somewhat	much	very much

4. My breathing rate increases

1	2	3	4	5
not at all	a little	somewhat	much	very much

5. I perspire

1	2	3	4	5
not at all	a little	somewhat	much	very much

FIGURE 4-5. Dental Fear Survey.

6. I feel nauseated and sick to my stomach

1	2	3	4	5
not at all	a little	somewhat	much	very much

7. My heart beats faster

1	2	3	4	5
not at all	a little	somewhat	much	very much

Following is a list of things and situations that many people mention as being somewhat anxiety or fear producing. Please rate how much fear, anxiety, or unpleasantness each of them causes you. Use the numbers 1–5, from the following scale. Make a check in the appropriate space. (If it helps, try to imagine yourself in each of these situations and describe what your common reaction is.)

1	2	3	4	5
not at all	a little	somewhat	much	very much

	1	2	3	4	5
8. Making an appointment for dentistry					
9. Approaching the dentist's office					
10. Sitting in the waiting room					
11. Being seated in the dental chair					
12. The smell of the dentist's office					
13. Seeing the dentist walk in					
14. Seeing the anesthetic needle					
15. Feeling the needle injected					
16. Seeing the drill					
17. Hearing the drill					
18. Feeling the vibrations of the drill					
19. Having your teeth cleaned					
20. All things considered, how fearful are you of having dental work done					

FIGURE 4-5. Continued.

In our research and clinical experience using this survey, we have found that most patients, whether fearful or not, have enjoyed being able to express their feelings concerning dentistry in this way. Many have reported that being given the opportunity to do so indicates to them that their dentist is interested in their personal well-being. Further, these responses provide a specific means by which dentists can begin or continue to discuss a patient's feelings.

DENTAL BELIEFS SURVEY

Most investigations into dental fear have focused on those technical procedures that patients most fear. However, as previously discussed, this presents only a partial picture of the concerns that are involved in a patient's fears. Little attention has been directed toward the subjective perceptions of the patient regarding the behavior of the dentist and the process of how the care is delivered. It was for this reason that the Dental Beliefs Survey (DBS) shown in Figure 4-6 was developed (Smith, Getz et al., 1984).

It is important to remember that the primary goal of the interview and the paper and pencil measures is to gain an understanding of the patients' perceptions concerning the reason for their fear. Thus the purpose of the DBS is to identify to what degree the patient perceives the behavior of the dental professional as being, or contributing to, the problem. Consequently, the information obtained is both diagnostic and prescriptive. The questions are designed to help you confirm your initial diagnostic impressions as well as suggest how you, as the health care provider, can tailor your approach to best address the specific concerns of the patient.

The survey questions patients about issues that are of primary concern to patients with General Anxiety or who are Distrustful. Because this survey was designed to complement the Dental Fear Survey, items pertaining to patients' physiological responses and specific stimuli were not included. There are four major areas of concern explored by this questionnaire: Communication, Belittlement, Lack of Power, and Trust.

NAME_____ SEX____ DATE _____

The items in this questionnaire refer to various situations, feelings, and re-actions related to dental work. Please rate your feeling or beliefs on these items by *circling the number* (1, 2, 3, 4, or 5) of the category which most closely corresponds to your feelings about dentists in general.

1. I do not think dentists like it when a patient makes a request.

1	2	3	4	5
never	a little	somewhat	often	nearly always

2. Dentists are efficient but it often seems they're in a hurry, so I feel rushed.

1	2	3	4	5
never	a little	somewhat	often	nearly always

When having dental work done:

3. I feel that dentists do not provide clear explanations.

1	2	3	4	5
never	a little	somewhat	often	nearly always

4. I feel that the dentists do not really listen to what I say.

1	2	3	4	5
never	a little	somewhat	often	nearly always

5. I feel the dentist will do what he wants, no matter what I might say I want.

1	2	3	4	5
never	a little	somewhat	often	nearly always

6. Dental professionals say things to make me feel guilty about the way I care for my teeth.

1	2	3	4	5
never	a little	somewhat	often	nearly always

7. I am not sure I can believe what the dentist says about the work that is needed.

1	2	3	4	5
never	a little	somewhat	often	nearly always

FIGURE 4-6. *Getz Dental Beliefs Survey.*

8. I think that dentists say things in a way to try and fool me.

1	2	3	4	5
never	a little	somewhat	often	nearly always

9. I feel that dentists do not take my worries (fears) seriously.

1	2	3	4	5
never	a little	somewhat	often	nearly always

10. I feel dentists put me down (make light of my fears).

1	2	3	4	5
never	a little	somewhat	often	nearly always

11. I worry if dentists are technically competent and do a good quality job.

1	2	3	4	5
never	a little	somewhat	often	nearly always

12. If I were to indicate that it hurts, I don't think the dentist will stop and try to correct the problem.

1	2	3	4	5
never	a little	somewhat	often	nearly always

13. When I am in the chair, I don't feel like I can stop the appointment for a rest, if I feel the need.

1	2	3	4	5
never	a little	somewhat	often	nearly always

14. I do not feel comfortable asking questions.

1	2	3	4	5
never	a little	somewhat	often	nearly always

15. The thought of "hearing all the bad news," or completing all the work needed could be enough to keep me from going for, or finishing treatment.

1	2	3	4	5
never	a little	somewhat	often	nearly always

FIGURE 4-6. Continued.

Communication

Extensive research in medicine has shown that a patient's perceived ease of communication is a critical variable in determining compliance with health care recommendations and satisfaction with services (Sackett and Haynes, 1976). We believe that communication is also a crucial variable in determining the degree to which a patient's fears are decreased or exacerbated. Scott et al. (1984) noted, for example, that highly anxious patients were reluctant to talk with the dentist.

Four questions (1, 3, 4, and 14) were included in the DBS to explore how well the patient believes the dentist communicates and how comfortable the patient feels in attempting to talk with the dentist. There are many reasons why patients might feel uncomfortable. For some, it may be that their childhood dentist was gruff and uncommunicative. For others it may be that the patient is not very "assertive" and has difficulty talking with people perceived as authority figures. Whatever its origins, it is you who must make the initial outreach to these patients. It is important with the non-communicative patient to repeatedly make statements such as, "If I say anything you do not understand, let me know" or "It's important for me to know how you are feeling." Also bear in mind that *how* you make these gestures is as important as *what* you actually say.

Question 15 focuses on a specific aspect of communication that has proven to be of importance in working with patients of our clinic. As mentioned previously, Gale (1972) found in his survey that the third most prevalent concern of fearful patients was the fear of "hearing bad news." Our data confirm this as one of the patient's chief concerns. This points out the extreme care with which information must be communicated, both following the initial examination and during the treatment plan presentaion. The issue of "bad news" presentation will be addressed in greater detail in Chapter 5.

Belittlement

Questions 6, 9, and 10 explore patients' beliefs or perceptions concerning how the dentist might view their fear and the condition of the teeth. Fear of belittlement is widespread. Hall and Edmondson (1983) note that "one of the commonest causes of dental fear has been shown to be anxiety lest the dentist should adopt a negative attitude. More than 61% of our patients indicate that they believe the dentist belittles or discounts their fears. And almost 71% of our patients feel that dental professionals are judgmental or make them feel guilty about their oral health."

Perhaps you feel these reports are exaggerated. They may be. And yet it is also very understandable. As a health professional, you know there is little to objectively fear. The procedures performed are seldom dangerous and in most cases are minimally painful. Thus we often attempt to reassure the patient that, "everything will be fine" or "it isn't that bad." Unfortunately, reassurance seldom works and patients often see it as a put-down. Similarly, because most health professonals *do* care about good health and their patients, it is easy to feel frustrated when patients act fearful, do not do what they are supposed to do, or when they neglect their health care. Consequently, difficulties can easily arise with a patient who is highly sensitized and frightened and who is ready to pick up on any indication of dentist frustration or disapproval. These tendencies are particularly strong in distrustful individuals.

Lack of Control or Power

As discussed in the preceding chapters, the issue of control is one of the major concerns of fearful patients. Approximately 86 percent of the patients we see indicate this is a critical issue for them. The following statements typify such patients' reports: "The dentist will do whatever he wants to, once he gets you in the chair." "I hate it when they hover over you." "They might as well be strapping you down—I feel pinned down." "I feel at their mercy." "They always take my glasses away so I can't tell what they are doing."

Being the expert on the technical aspects of dental treatment, you do not consult the patient on how to perform a MOD on #30. Consequently, it is very easy to ignore working with the patient to encourage his or her participation in treatment, which in turn might give the patient the perception of having no control or power. Questions 5, 12, and 13 examine the patients' beliefs about their ability to control what goes on during a typical treatment. At first glance, it may be difficult to believe that a patient does not feel that he or she could stop an appointment if in severe pain. And yet, this fear is frequently identified by patients as their primary concern.

As you might guess, many patients lack skills in self-assertion. Upon questioning, you will learn that they have difficulty making requests for fear of disapproval by the dentist or the hygienist. They are likely to "sit there and take it," vowing not to return because "I can't stand the thought of going back." You will note that only question 11 relates to the patient's beliefs concerning the dentist's technical skills. Contrary to our initial expectations, we found that only a small minority of patients worry about the dentist's technical competence. Although they may be terrified of dentistry, they seldom are very concerned about the dentist "bungling it." The exceptions are generally patients who have experienced traumatic incidents in the chair such as profuse bleeding caused by an obvious operator error.

Trust

The issue of trust is addressed by two questions of the DBS (7 and 8). In our patients, we find approximately 12 percent mark these affirmatively. Obviously, the more skeptical or distrustful the patient is initially, the more difficult he or she is to treat. Such patients are not ready to accept or put faith in your good intentions or reassurances. These patients are often angry and concerned that you may deceive them.

PATIENTS WITH SIGNIFICANT PSYCHOLOGICAL PROBLEMS

At this point we wish to discuss those patients who present a seemingly jumbled, complex or extreme picture of some of the conditions and beliefs discussed previously. There are some patients who are simply too difficult for the average practitioner to successfully work with. The purpose of this section is to help you recognize and screen such patients, rather than how to treat them. These individuals are best treated in conjunction with a psychotherapist or psychologist who has had experience with this type of patient. Such patients will almost always fall within the Generalized Anxiety and Catastrophe categories and will be extremely fearful. It will often be difficult for you to keep the patient to the point as they jump around relating seemingly disconnected events. For example, you may find an individual who has a strong fear of being alone in crowds, unfamiliar places, driving, bridges, or closed spaces where "help" may not be available in case of sudden incapacitation. This patient is generally accompanied to the office by a relative or friend and is most likely to be a non-employed woman who to some degree appears house-bound. This cluster of symptoms may be a sign of a condition known as *agoraphobia* (DSM III, 1980). Studies estimate that approximately 0.5 percent of the population has this condition at some time. Periods of remission are common. This patient generally has a series of panic attacks and becomes reluctant to place himself or herself in any situation that might trigger these events. Dentistry is often such a trigger. Although they tend to ascribe their problems to physiology, they seldom have such episodes when they are on familiar ground where they tend to feel safe.

Another type of patient you may see are the severely depressed. Your first indication may be the medical history form where they list prescription drugs being taken. That is not to say that every patient who comes in taking Valium® or Elavil® is severely depressed. It does, however, indicate an avenue to explore further. What are the symptoms of the severely depressed? The patient will talk about what he or she "should" do, but expresses doubts about wanting to, or ability to do anything. There is a feeling of "What good will it do," of "hopelessness," or a response of "I guess that would be nice" in a flat, almost defeated tone.

A third type of patient who is difficult to work with is the patient who appears to sincerely, almost desperately, wish to succeed in getting dental work done, but who finds almost everything in life overwhelming and incapacitating. They may talk about "getting their life together," but appear so paralyzed with anxiety and fear they can make no positive step.

What should you do when confronted with this type of individual? If the patient is already in psychotherapy or counseling, we suggest that you ask permission to contact his or her therapist or counselor. For example, you might say, "From what you have said, dentistry appears to be a difficult area to deal with. My goal is to be able to provide you the dental treatment you need—at the same time structuring it so that it will not be a traumatic experience for you. Because I want this to be a positive experience for you I would like to consult with your therapist about how I might best treat you. Do I have your permission to call?"

For those patients who are not currently seeing a counselor you might say, "In talking with you, you have mentioned a large number of concerns of which coping with dentistry is only one. In other words, there are other situations in which these problems come up. It might be helpful for you to see a counselor who could help you learn how to better handle these situations. What you learn could then be applied to the specific problem of receiving dental care as well as the other issues you raised. Are you interested?"

In summary, there are some situations and patients whose problems are too involved for you to treat successfully. Your best alternative is to refer the patient to a more skilled clinician or possibly a psychological counselor. Appendix B talks about how to find and select a psychological professional.

UTILIZING EXISTING RECORDS TO ASSESS FEARFUL PATIENTS

We have saved this section for last because it is the most indirect method for ascertaining if a patient is fearful. In addition, its usefulness is, to a large degree, dependent upon the quality of the charting system. A chart without notations regarding patient behavior or an accurate record of cancellations will obviously be of less use than those more complete notes.

Over a period of time, every practice accumulates a number of patients who are "goers but haters"; individuals who fail to respond to recall notices; or are "irregular appointment makers"; or patients who too fre-

145

quently cancel or fail to show up for an appointment. There are of course many different reasons for patients presenting behavior problems. However, anxiety and fear about dentistry are frequently major inhibiting factors, and, as noted earlier, some patients are reluctant to openly express their fear to the dentist or auxiliaries.

As was described previously, the record of appointments made and kept or missed can serve as a cue to alert the dentist to possible problems of fear. Bernstein, Kleinknecht and Alexander (1979) reported that patients previously identified as fearful through a questionnaire mailed to them were six times more likely to cancel or not appear for a given appointment than were persons who reported not being fearful. Cancellation of appointments, of course, can occur for a variety of reasons in addition to fearfulness. Records of appointment changes or a sporadic irregular distribution with two or more years between appointments can serve as an initial sign of fearfulness, but, of course, must be supported by additional information.

Another indicator of possible fearfulness, obtainable from records, is the patient's having had a long history of chronic illness. In many cases, lengthy histories of illness and possibly painful and traumatic treatment can leave one sensitized to all settings of a medical nature. This is particularly true if the patient is a child. The similiarity of the dental office and routine might appear to such patients as one more situation in which they will receive painful injections or other traumatic treatments. On the other hand, some such chronically ill patients, through their many medical experiences, may have become indifferent to treatment and not react at all. Nonetheless, the patient's previous medical history might serve as another indicator and is worth the small amount of time it takes to make this observation.

A third source of information from records are clinical notes concerning a patient's behavior from previous appointments. This, of course, can be of value only if the dentist or an assistant takes the time to record his or her impressions following an appointment. Such notation is particularly important when we consider that many patients come for treatment or examinations at several years' intervals. One's memory cannot be counted on to remember each patient, especially those who have not been in for several years. Further, behavioral impressions, regularly noted, can provide evidence of patient change over time.

Information gathered from patient records can serve as the basis for development of the hypothesis concerning the patient's level of fearfulness, which can then be followed up in more detail from subsequent sources of information. We will discuss how to make useful behavioral notes regarding patient behavior at a later point.

The first step is to review the patient's files to identify "problem" patients—those who are difficult to work with in the chair, and those patients who have failed to follow through a treatment or regular preventive appointments. We have found that it can be very effective if the dentist personally makes reactivation calls. However, in most offices, this task will be assigned to the office receptionist.

If a staff person is to make the call, he or she should be briefed on the procedure to follow when he or she contacts the patient. As we will repeatedly stress, if a dentist chooses to work with the fearful patient, the entire staff must be brought aboard. Successful treatment requires a team approach.

Upon reaching a patient by phone, a conversation might go something like this:

Staff: Mrs. Roberts, this is Ann from Dr. Humphries' office. We were going through our files and realized that we haven't seen you in a year and a half. Dr. Humphries asked me to call you about making an appointment.

Patient: Well, I had been thinking about it. I just hadn't gotten around to it. I'm a little short of cash right now. I've been real busy . . . etc.

Staff: Well, I can certainly understand how that could get in the way. Dentistry is certainly an easy thing to delay. Some people I find would rather do almost anything to avoid going to the dentist. Are you a person who has to force herself to go?

Patient: Yeah, I really don't like it much.

Staff: Because it is uncomfortable and/or scary?

Patient: Oh I know it's kind of crazy but I always get nervous thinking about it.

Staff: Oh, in that case I am glad I called. Dr. Humphries is very concerned with his patients, especially those who are nervous about going to the dentist. If you would like to make an appointment, I will make a note for Dr. Humphries to meet with you in his office to discuss with you what it is he can do to make it as easy as possible for you to receive care. May we set up an appointment?

With some simple telephone techniques you are more than simply increasing your business level. You are communicating a clear message to your patients that you are concerned about their health, listening to them, and providing service.

CONCLUSION

We have now examined the process of how to go about making a diagnosis of the fearful patient.

As was mentioned in the beginning of this chapter, there is no one single sign of behavior that will point to a definite diagnosis. Each piece of information collected must be placed in context with every other to gradually form a picture of the problem. It is for this reason that we emphasize that each person in the office has a role as an observer, from the time the receptionist first speaks with the patient on the telephone and on through the treatment appointments. Your task is to find the answers to two questions: What is the patient actually afraid of? How does the patient respond to the fear? The interview questions, observation of the signs of anxiety, and the paper and pencil questionnaires are simply tools to help you answer those questions. With a working understanding of the four types of fear, the pieces of the puzzle can be placed together to help you reach a diagnosis and select the treatment strategies that have the highest probability of being successful. Diagnosis is an inexact science at best. However, with practice, as with any other skill, our accuracy improves. And what if you initially misdiagnose, or choose a strategy which seemingly does not work? The same rules and procedures apply in this area as they do in any other; you ask further questions, reanalyze what you have already obtained, and try the next strategy.

The four types of fear patients discussed here were (1) fear of specific stimuli, (2) distrust of dental personnel, (3) generalized anxiety, and (4) fear of catastrophe.

QUESTIONS AND EXERCISES

1. Describe two main differences between patients fearful of catastrophe and those with generalized anxiety.

2. Describe several signs of fear which the dentist or auxiliaries can *observe* prior to and during treatment. For each of these signs, what reasons other than fear might be responsible for their occurrence? How might you determine if they are caused by fear or by other factors? Observe your next patient and evaluate the presence and/or degree of each of these signs.

3. Have your next patients complete the Dental Fear Survey and Dental Beliefs Scale. How many would you predict have ever put off making an appointment due to fear? How many would you predict have ever canceled an appointment due to fear? Record the patients' responses and evaluate the differences from your predictions. If there are differences, how do you account for them?

4. What types of patients are more likely to be identified by the Dental Beliefs Survey rather than by the Dental Fears Survey? What are the differences between them?

5. After your patients have completed the Dental Fears Survey and the Dental Beliefs Scale, ask them how they felt about completing these forms. Did they find it of interest, an annoyance? Also, ask them if they think it would be a good idea to have patients routinely fill them out.

FIVE

Practice Management with Fearful Patients

In this chapter we discuss general strategies useful with every patient. The chapter is organized into the following sections: examination and treatment planning; emergencies: scheduling and finances; and home care. Chapters 6–9 present specialized treatment techniques appropriate for specific types of fear.

THE INITIAL EXAMINATION

From a dental standpoint, the purpose of the exam is to obtain an accurate picture of the individual's overall dental health and reach a tentative diagnosis. From a patient management perspective, the exam has three primary functions:

1. To present information in a positive manner in order to mitigate the fear of receiving "bad news."

2. To let patients know they will be consulted and listened to regarding treatment preferences.

3. To demonstrate to patients they will not be surprised or be "forced" to do anything against their will.

It is important to remember that during the initial examination your words and gestures are being scrutinized very closely. At this point patients try to determine if you are really different from other dentists and dental personnel they have known. Because the dental environment is so familiar to us, we forget that to many patients dentistry is mysterious or threatening. Consequently, the *overall rule* is inform the patient what it is you wish to do, what the purpose is, and ask if it is "ok" to proceed.

Conduct procedures in order of priority. The longer the exam process, the greater the anxiety most fearful patients will experience. Thus, proceed to gather essential information: the condition of carious or damaged teeth or periodontal condition of key areas of the mouth. Reserve the "nice-to-know" aspects of the exam such as periodontal probings of all the teeth or condition of asymptomatic third molars for another visit. These data may be important but are best gathered when more rapport is established with the patient. Painful tests, such as electric pulp testing, can be carried out after reviewing radiographs. For many highly fearful patients, your initial exam may have to be conducted visually without explorer or probe. Only when trust is established can you gain permission to use these other instruments. Avoid using air syringes or water in these patients. If the teeth are covered in plaque, use a wet 2x2 cotton gauze and gently wipe the teeth. Your gentleness will be appreciated by the prospective patient.

Presenting Information: The Good News-Bad News Dilemma

As we discussed in Chapter 1, Gale (1972) reported that the third most common fear mentioned by patients was that of "hearing bad news." Our clinical experience supports this finding. At times fears are very specific: "I know the dentist will find all my teeth have to be extracted," or "all my expensive crowns are failing." Clearly the examination appointment will be stressful for these patients. Other patients, though not fearing a specific calamity, are convinced—usually because they have not seen the dentist in a few years—that "the doctor will find something horribly wrong with me." Their imaginations run wild during a routine exam. Imagining that everything written down is "another problem," such patients can become so anxious that by the time you are ready to explain what you have found, they cannot listen to what you have to say.

Vocabulary is also important. Highly technical vocabulary is of no use to the patient and certain terms (e.g., root canal) are often very poorly understood and frightening. At the same time, pedodontic terms (e.g., "putting the tooth to sleep") may be perceived as patronizing and may breed distrust. Our experience is that you should use lay terms as much as possible and avoid detailed explanations. To the extent explanations are necessary, there will be time later after a therapeutic relationship is established. It is important to remember that fear, like any other intense emotion, impedes our ability to listen to a message. We still hear the words, but our "perceptual filters" change and selectively screen out parts of the message. We routinely begin the examination by trying to explain what we are doing. Imagine the following conversation:

Dentist: I want to take a thorough look at your teeth and gums to learn about what's going on in there. To do that I want to use my little mirror and explorer. Is that ok with you?

Patient: Yeah, but don't stick it in my teeth—especially in the back on top!

Dentist: O.K. I will be careful. While I do this I will ask Jane, my assistant, to write down information, so that I can make a map of your mouth. Most of what I will say will be about work that has already been done—in other words it won't all be bad news! After I'm done I will explain to you in "English" what I find and you can ask questions. Are you ready to begin?

Such an explanation helps reduce the patient's fears. It lets him know a time to talk and ask questions will follow the exam. We encourage patients who are obviously fearful to bring a friend or relative to the office to accompany them into the operatory for the exam. The friend may be able to "listen better" than the anxious person, and frequently act as a strong supporter afterwards in encouraging the patient to proceed with treatment.

Asking Permission

You will note in the previous conversation that the dentist asked twice if what was proposed was "OK" with the patient. We do not ask these questions rhetorically. The use of this technique allows you to accomplish two patient management objectives: letting the patient know he will be consulted, and that there will be "no surprises." Asking permission allows the patient to feel that he or she has a role in treatment. Frequently patients feel that they do not know what is going on, and have no right to participate or comment about the preferences for treatment. The importance of this is clear when you consider how people act when they are afraid. Fear makes an individual hesitant to "go ahead" with the frightening event. Thus, a person who feels he or she is "being pushed" may find a way to resist. We have encountered numerous patients who have failed to return to other dentists for treatment after being "frightened to death" about the work needed. Or having returned, they refuse to begin treatment. Similarly, many practitioners have expressed their frustration about spending hour-long appointments without success trying to persuade a patient to proceed.

Asking permission places the responsibility for treatment with the patient. You may question: "Don't patients abuse this privilege? Who's in charge here, me or the patient?" Recall, from Chapter 4, one of the most common fears is being helpless and under the control of the dentist. We have all been taught to check during treatment with a patient, "How are you doing?" In the same way, asking permission is checking to see if the patient is ready to proceed. It enhances the patient's control, and has the paradoxical effect of allowing progress more quickly than if you tried to push the patient.

Concluding the Initial Examination

At this point you should explain your tentative conclusions. Because of our professional training, most of us begin by listing the most severe problems found. For example, a dentist might begin by saying: "The primary problem is this tooth that hurts. It looks like you will need a root canal, which is a procedure where we take out the nerve and replace it with an inert plug. You have two new cavities that need to be filled, and a few old fillings that should be replaced. You also have moderate periodontal disease which will require treatment. This may sound like a lot of work, but it is all pretty routine dentistry, and everything should turn out 'OK' by the time we finish."

What is wrong with this approach? First, it focuses exclusively on what is *wrong*. Secondly, it begins by mentioning the need for a root canal, one of the most feared procedures in dentistry. With this beginning, the probability has increased dramatically that your patient will not remember half of what is said and may not return. Also, for some patients, the implied cost (psychic and financial) may be overwhelming.

Compare the above with the following: "Let me begin by saying that most of your teeth are in good shape. You have two kinds of problems—both of which can be successfully treated. I'm glad you came in now, rather than waiting longer. We can make you healthy again. The problem I am most concerned with is the infection in your gums. It is the infection which makes your teeth so sensitive, and the problem which can eventually cause more problems than anything else.

"The second problem involves your teeth. There are two new cavities and two to three old fillings that need to be repaired. All of them involve routine patch work and they will be 'good as new' after we're done. The last tooth I want to discuss is the one that you pointed out as bothering you. Although I need to do some more tests, it looks as though that tooth will need more complicated treatment, which I will explain in detail later. It too should turn out fine. I want to give you some antibiotics to reduce the infection in that tooth (which also will help the gums). Also, I'd like to start with some simpler procedures so that I can get to know how you react to treatment, and you have a chance to get to know me. Do you have any questions?"

In summary, your task is to let the patient know what is "OK" about his health, and present the problems in a non-overwhelming way so that the patient can understand that there is a solution. Specific details about the various treatments can be provided shortly prior to or in conjunction with the treatment itself.

The Case Consultation

Except for very simple cases, we have each patient return for a consultation appointment. This allows us to carefully examine the information collected and plan out how we wish to proceed. During this appointment we repeat much of what was said following the initial examination, adding to the outline the specific treatments proposed, including possible alternatives, and the time and cost involved. It is helpful to prioritize phases of treatment and set goals. For example, if the patient is now symptomatic, you can briefly describe the plan for getting the patient more comfortable and beginning to stabilize his condition. If, on the other hand, he needs regular preventive care, you can describe this without extensive discussion of rehabilitation. Goals should be set for short (e.g., three–six month) manageable periods. For example, "We'll treat your periodontal condition now and in three months re-evaluate your restorative needs." As with any patient, use the consultation with the fearful patient as an opportunity to educate and motivate. Use the mirror, X-rays, or models to demonstrate the conditions you are focusing on. Avoid abstract concepts. Also avoid long laundry lists of treatment needed. Summarize rather than describe every procedure to be accomplished. Instead, offer the patient a written treatment plan and estimate to take home. This is helpful also because others may be involved in the treatment or financial aspects of the case.

Treatment Planning

How do you decide where to begin? Should you, for example, always start with getting the patient cleaned up, moving then next to the most serious dental problems, and leaving the cosmetic work until the end? Which should come first, periodontal treatment or restorative treatment? Our experience has led us to the conclusion that treatment planning for the fearful patient must be flexible. The order needs to be determined by what the patient finds fearful and what the patient considers important.

For example, with a patient terrified of pain, a gingival infection may be initially treated with antibiotics and repeated coronal polishing. This will establish trust and desensitize the patient to the dental environment as well as improve the gums. Another patient may be embarrassed by what he or she perceives as "horrible looking front teeth." In this case you might begin by restoring the anteriors with composite. The procedures are simple and results good. In one patient recently, we began by realigning anteriors with an orthodontic appliance. We felt we could not place attractive composites until we did this. The result was a very grateful patient who had never before considered that his teeth could look so nice. This can be done even if future treatment may involve crowns or endodontics.

What might you say to the patient when it becomes clear that the patient's priorities differ from yours? Imagine the following conversation.

Dentist: From talking with you I understand that getting your front teeth looking better is very important to you.

Patient: Yes, if I could only do that I would feel much better.

Dentist: From my viewpoint, I feel that some of your other problems are more serious. You are likely to develop a toothache if I don't take care of the back teeth first. My preference would be to treat those first. However, I am willing to do what you want as long as you know what could happen. What do you think?

This approach places the responsibility and decision with the patient. He or she chooses and thus is involved in the process. Attempting too early in treatment to persuade the patient to do what you think the patient should do can establish a *push-resist* relationship.

Another clinical problem we often see is the endodontically involved, severely damaged anterior tooth. This is a high priority because of the esthetics. Our approach is to take out the pulp, debride and medicate the canal, and place a temporary post and acrylic crown. Making this tooth the focus of attention also allows us to get the patient cleaning around the front tooth!

Still another clinical problem is found in teeth requiring extraction. With the patient's permission, we will often wait to extract hopeless teeth until after other priorities are met. We have found that although there may be flareups, patients blame the pain on the tooth, not on the dentist, as long as prompt steps are taken when this occurs. Extractions are not positive steps because they do not create better looking teeth and they are considered painful by many patients. Consider putting them lower on the list of priorities with the patient's permission.

How about procedures involving injections? As discussed in Chapter 3, we believe dentists *under use* local anesthetic. Nonetheless, for the injection-resistant patient, several short visits for coronal polish or simple supragingival scaling may be indicated. Consider restoring a non-vital tooth.

One final point about treatment planning. We have observed that many dentists *under treat* fearful patients because they are difficult. Our experience suggests that careful planning will result in a patient who is relatively easy to care for and is maintained in practice for many years. At the same time, assume that the patient will be around for many years and save some less immediate care (elective crowns, posterior bridges, etc.) for a follow-up period. Consider terminating the initial phase of treatment as follows:

Dentist: I am extremely pleased with your progress. All the holes you came in with are repaired and your gums are healthy.

Patient: Yes, I am really happy with how things have gone. I wouldn't have done this with any other dentist.

Dentist: Thank you. When I see you in three months for a checkup on your gums, we need to begin to talk about making you a really nice crown for your front tooth. You can think about it in the meantime and we can talk about it then.

EMERGENCIES

Fearful patients have more emergencies than those who are non-fearful. This is because they avoid care and do not practice adequate self-care. Chronic avoiders frequently have badly broken down teeth and acute endodontic and periodontic lesions. Pain probably will bring them in and provides an opportunity to break the chain of symptomatic treatment.

Several general rules are helpful. First, be available. Return emergency telephone calls promptly and do not delay scheduling appointments. Second, use the first few minutes to establish rapport. Only if the patient sees you (and your staff) as non-judgmental and truly supportive will the patient return. Finally, try hard to use medications (analgesics, long-acting anesthetics, and antibiotics) to get over the acute phase. If at all possible, avoid operative or surgical treatment at the time the patient is in pain. If you do not, you probably will hurt the patient.

Instead, as suggested in Chapter 3, long-acting anesthetics injected locally (e.g., 1.8–3.6 ml bupivacaine 0.5% with 1:200,000 epinephrine) can provide up to 12 hours relief for pulpitis (Moore and Dunstay, 1983). Our experience is that this with analgesics (e.g., aspirin–30 mg codeine) can provide enough relief for the patient to sleep and calm down. The effects of antibiotics are slower and less predictable, especially for inflamed pulps. Nonetheless, use of the penicillins for pulpitis (Accepted Dental Therapeutics, 1982) or tetracyclines for periodontal abscesses (Marder and Milgrom, 1984) is recommended. Consider 1 week, 250–500 mg four times per day.

If you need to go ahead and open a tooth or debride an abscess for emergency purposes, do everything you can not to traumatize the patient. First, do not give long, scary explanations. Keep it simple. Second, use lots of anesthetic. Try to eliminate as much pain as possible. Third, allow for frequent rest breaks—every few minutes ask the patient to stand up and sip some fruit juice. Finally, be supportive and let the patient know everything will turn out ok. Try not to appear rushed and avoid anger and put-downs if the patient has trouble with the visit. Finally, be sure to do a careful differential diagnosis before you begin. Fearful patients will report colorful symptoms. Sinus or muscle pain may be reported as unbearable tooth pain and, for the unwary clinician, result in unnecessary endodontics or surgical treatment for the patient.

SCHEDULING APPOINTMENTS

Length

In scheduling, it is natural to think primarily in terms of the technical procedures to be performed and how long it normally takes to complete them. Consequently, appointment length is conceived as revolving around our convenience, not the patient's preference. In working with the fearful patient, take a different approach. We almost invariably schedule the first few appointments for 20 to 40 minutes maximum. We do this for three reasons. First, we tell the patient that we will want to begin slowly so that he or she can begin to get to know who we are and become more comfortable.

Second, by scheduling short appointments, we can accomplish a small task and praise the patient for succeeding. We want the patient to feel that each appointment was successful and that he or she *could* have gone on longer. Our goal is to avoid having the patient say to himself, "I made it through, but I could never go back."

Finally, if the patient *does* encounter difficulties, you do not suddenly find yourself left with a huge block of unproductive time because he could not go on any longer. This strategy also minimizes scheduling disruptions if a patient cancels or fails. Some patients feel as if they should be able to "take it" and will push themselves. As described in Chapters 6 and 9, patients who "attempt to be brave" are most often afraid of aversive stimuli or catastrophe. With these patients, especially in the beginning, it is the clinician who has to put limits on how long the appointment will be. However, there are other patients, particulary the anxious individual described in Chapter 8, who eventually may have to be pushed to increase their appointment length. While many non-fearful patients might find it annoying to have short appointments and come more frequently, we have found that most fearful patients find it easier to cope with a shorter treatment session. How can dental work be structured in order to make this feasible? There are times when it takes some creativity. However, it is more often simply a matter of thinking about the problem differently. For example:

Very Short Procedures

Coronal polish, one quadrant

Alginate impressions, one arch

Polish a filling

Supragingival scaling, one quadrant

Home care instruction, upper or lower anteriors

Short Procedures

Ultrasonic scaling

Class I, III, V fillings

Scale one quadrant

Pit and fissure sealants

Fluoride treatment, one arch

Temporary filling

Nonetheless, it's important to let the patient participate in deciding how to proceed. The choice of procedure will vary. Obviously, someone afraid of gagging is not a candidate for an initial impression.

Intervals Between Appointments

This appears to be a highly individual preference. Some patients find that once started that they are willing to come in twice a week. Others prefer every other week. We have found, however, that any larger interval than this tends to allow the anxiety about dentistry to begin to build up once again. If an extended period of time goes by without an appointment you should expect some relapse in the patient's coping skills. Be prepared to start on something easy again even if he has progressed significantly prior to the lapse. Two other considerations are important. For some patients it is necessary to demonstrate a progression of improvement—in gum health or attractive anterior fillings. Long intervals make it difficult to keep temporaries in place and infected teeth out of pain or gums healthy.

Appointment Keeping/Cancellation

Late patients, last-minute cancellations, and failures are the bane of all practices. This is a problem that is especially frequent with fearful patients. Interestingly, the highest rate of failures in our clinic occurs with those individuals who make an initial appointment but fail to appear. You will recall from Chapter 4 that during the initial interview we ask patients if they are the kind of person who is likely to fail or cancel appointments. This information appears to be generally predictive of failure behavior and helps us determine who will receive the majority of our appointment confirmation efforts. Because of the problem with initial appointments, this may be a question to be asked over the phone when the appointment is made. We find it appropriate to ask these patients for suggestions on how to get them to show up. Frequently patients suggest telephone reminders. In addition, we keep records on lateness and failures and cancellations. An attempt to identify these patients as quickly as possible will reduce the economic and emotional consequences of the problem.

The largest percentage of failures and cancellations occurs with a small minority of patients. There are two principal reasons for appointment failure. The first is fear of treatment. It has been our experience that this fades following three to four visits. The second reason, however, is more indicative of the patient's style rather than a result of specific dental fear. As a general rule, persons falling within the generalized anxiety category (see Chapter 8) are more likely to exhibit a pattern where conflicts, emotional traumas, and "circumstances" get in the way of making the dental appointment or almost any other commitment to be at a given place at a given time.

This problem is illustrated by a patient seen by one of our students in the restorative dentistry clinic. The student sought help because the patient was chronically 30 minutes to one hour late for visits. The problem occurred in the morning and afternoon and was resistant to exhortations on the health value of treatment and to the student's anger. The diagnosis was unrecognized anxiety. Greater patient control over the length and type of appointments, mutual recognition, and an empathic response by the student dentist reduced the problem to manageable proportions.

For the patient whose coping style involves failing appointments, a different strategy may be helpful. One approach we occasionally use is especially good for those individuals who profess that they want to come for regular treatment but, without pain, lack motivation. It is called "donation to the most hated organization." We ask the patient to identify a hated organization or political candidate and request that he or she write out a check for $50 or more to the organization or campaign. The patient is told the address of the organization will be located and that the check will be mailed if he or she does not meet the commitment. We ask if this would be sufficient motivation for them to show up. We note parenthetically that not only would they be supporting an organization that they despised, but that they would now be on the organization's mailing list. If considered subversive, they may also be on the FBI's list as well. At this point most patients agree that the consequences of this strategy will ensure attendance.

Another more conventional approach that is helpful is appointment follow-up calls. Sometimes our impression of a previous visit is more positive than that of the patient. Their negative evaluation may cause appointment failure. Such a case is illustrated here.

A 40-year-old female had originally visited our clinic about one year ago. She had previously avoided care for over six years and was afraid of being hurt and put down for the condition of her teeth. She was treated successfully and put on recall. She returned for the scheduled appointment. At this time it was noted that she had stopped her previously fastidious oral hygiene habits; she reported being afraid a crown would come off if she cleaned around it. She had a periodontal abscess and aggravated gingivitis. The abscess was treated with closed curettage and antibiotics. A second appointment was scheduled. The problem responded well *and efforts were made to desensitize her fears "about cleaning too hard."* She was placed on a more frequent recall schedule, but failed her next appointment. Much to the chagrin of the clinician, a follow-up call from the psychologist found she had felt "put-down" because of the way he handled the abscess. While the patient responded normally in the operatory, she failed her next appointment. A follow-up call right after the appointment would have revealed the problem.

It is best, from our experience, to make a definite appointment for the future while the patient is present in the office. Also, the phone is much better than a letter or card.

A final suggestion is to try having some patients confirm their own appointments. Here we give patients cards with the telephone number and ask them to call us to hold their place. This reduces the burden on our staff and gives some patients a mechanism to accept responsibility.

There is no pat answer to the appointment control problem. We suggest you employ several methods with difficult patients and avoid showing anger. If you find it impossible to continue scheduling the patient, keep the door open. Tell him you will be glad to see him in the future when he is able to make his appointments more regularly. Our observation is that some patients view an appointment like an airline reservation. You can cancel if it suits you. For such patients, we ask for a deposit through the mail (say $50) to confirm their appointment. If they show, we apply it to their bill; if not, it becomes a non-refundable charge.

FINANCES

As with any other population, this is a recurrent problem. Interestingly, the proportion of our patients with some kind of dental insurance is similar to that of the general population in our area. Financial need is not the primary barrier for most of our patients.

This is not to say, however, that financial factors are not a consideration. Because so many of our patients have avoided care for long periods, there is often extensive work needed. Consequently, even for those individuals with insurance their portion of the bill is often substantial. In addition, most dental plans will not pay for the psychological services that are part of our treatment protocol. How then do we handle patient finances?

You will remember that we stated that we begin treatment, and to a large extent continue, at a pace that most practices would consider very slow. This is done as a deliberate treatment strategy. It also has consequences for practice management. The fact that we move slowly means that the work and the costs are spread over an extended period. Consequently, we can more easily work out a payment plan that both we and the patient can live with.

PREVENTION: ORAL SELF-CARE

Home Care

While most of this book attempts to help the dental care team provide successful dental treatment experiences for fearful patients, the long term prognosis for all patients is poor if they do not routinely practice a minimal level of oral self-care.

Some of our fearful patients have, without professional assistance for years, developed and adhered to an adequate regimen. These patients, albeit a minority, are consciously trying to compensate for a lack of professional supervision. They eagerly accept information that will help them enhance the effectiveness and efficiency of their regimens. Maintaining optimal oral health based on a concern of the consequences of neglect can be appropriate. On the other hand, the vast majority of such patients either do not maintain a daily regimen of oral self-care and/or clean superficially or ineffectively. Many of these individuals have disease-ravaged mouths that give new meaning to the "bombed out" metaphor. Such mouths are difficult and painful to clean. One can imagine the downward spiral of avoidance of care, deterioration and decay, difficulty of self-care, and subsequent deterioration of health.

Competent health professionals in many disciplines are frequently stymied when they present preventive or therapeutic regimens—either prescriptions or proscriptions for patient behavior. Even when the prescription is easily within their power, e.g., taking a pill, many patients do not comply with professional advice. Researchers believe 30 to 70 percent of *all* recommendations for home care, medication, diet, or exercise are not complied with by patients. A 50 percent rate of noncompliance in self-reported frequency of brushing or flossing (or both) has emerged as the high-water mark of success in primary preventive activities with normal dental patients. The enormity of the problem is staggering, especially when periodontitis and caries are controllable with the cooperation of patients. The problem is greater with fearful patients.

Though dentists and hygienists in the 1960s and early 1970s responded enthusiastically to new scientific findings by promoting plaque control, by the mid 1970s enthusiasm faded because programs failed to produce successful long-term outcomes. Studies showed a regression to the initial levels of home care behavior. This research has shown that even patients who initially follow new home care instruction do not maintain the behavior without intermittent professional supervision.

On the other hand, the emergence of a new behavioral medicine specialty called Behavioral Health has presented us with new promise. This discipline focuses on the application of behavioral and biomedical science knowledge and techniques to the maintenance of health and prevention of illness and dysfunction by a variety of self-initiated or shared activities. Many studies enhancing exercise, diet management, and a variety of other long-term health behaviors have been reported, some of which have occurred in dentistry. Weinstein, Fiset, and Lancaster (1984) reviewed this literature and reported the long-term successfulness of a behavioral plaque program. Weinstein, Getz, and Milgrom (1984) describe the steps of this program in detail in their handbook. Over the last few years considerable data have been collected that point to the effectiveness of this approach.

The next few pages specify basic behavioral principles necessary in plaque control. These are especially important in working with fearful patients.

Plaque Control

COMMUNICATION IS CRITICAL. Considerable care must be taken when plaque control programs are introduced. The way in which patients are introduced to an oral self-care program may greatly influence their decision to agree to alter their present habits.

Many patients believe they are already doing an acceptable job of cleaning their teeth. Some patients may have even felt slighted or coerced by comments and suggestions that intimate that they are incompetent in oral self-care. Care must be taken when plaque control is introduced because the criticism of present care habits can be implied by simply raising the topic.

Although customary, the initial hygiene appointment is not the best time to introduce plaque control techniques. A non-individualized approach may cause difficulties for plaque control programs, especially with fearful, distrustful patients. To influence the patient's thinking and action, the dentist, hygienist, and assistant must be aware of the dental needs and goals of the patient. It is often assumed that when the patient understands the cause of the disease and the effectiveness of preventive health practice, behavior will change. However, the research firmly indicates that information does not lead to altered behavior. Almost all children, by the time they reach the seventh grade, have heard that smoking is dangerous to their health, and yet, by this time, approximately 20 percent are already smoking. Old myths die hard.

Gold (1974) notes that many dentists who tell their patients about plaque control are often unaware that how they are relating to the patient is more important than what they are relating. The how of the doctor-patient interaction is the process of communication. The act of motivating a patient involves showing concern, listening, and providing information. Listening skills are critical, as is the expression of personal concerns. Patients may judge concern by the amount of time the professional spends listening and discussing the patients' problems. Information has a secondary role in motivating patients.

ASSESS READINESS. At a given point, many individuals are not willing to consider altering their present self-care patterns, and some may never be ready. Dentist or hygienist pressure may result in a superficial acquiescence, and the patient may even attempt to try the new self-care behavior. However, the probability of creating a long-term change is minimal.

It is useful to identify fearful patients who are likely or unlikely to respond to efforts to alter their existing self-care behavior. Patients who are likely to respond can be introduced to plaque control; alternate procedures, frequent recall prophylaxes, and fluorides, for example, can be discussed with those who are unlikely to respond to the plaque control approach.

There has been little research in dentistry that attempted to identify those who are ready to alter self-care habits. However, there is some evidence that a history of an active role in maintaining health, e.g., exercise regimes, controlled diet/nutrition, or control or elimination of smoking, is a positive predictor. The stated intent of the patient to change when questioned is also useful. In all, when the patient perceives that he or she has a problem, and has a preventive orientation ("holistic" is a trendy term used to describe such health-consciousness) or a history of careful self-care, he is ready to alter sub-optimal patterns of dental cleaning. We find fearful patients who have just made the crucial decision to seek dental care are often very good candidates for home care instruction.

SKILL LEVEL. Careful assessment of existing patient self-care practice is important. Although plaque control instruction often focuses on skill training, dentists and auxiliaries often do not systematically evaluate patient skills *before* instruction. This is a little more time-consuming, but the effort is invaluable when the instruction is being tailored to the patient's needs.

Knowledge of how the patient cleans his or her teeth at home can only come from observation of the patient's skills. It is our experience that, when asked to demonstrate skills, a patient will attempt to perform optimally, spending much time and effort to clean. As the patient attempts to avoid embarrassment, awkward and unfamiliar manipulations of instruments may become evident. When skills are being assessed, it should be stressed that you are interested in seeing this "at home" routine and that a showing of extraordinary effort in optimal cleansing is not useful.

The demonstration of routine "at home" self-care practices often discloses serious deficiencies. The lingual surfaces are the areas most commonly omitted during toothbrushing. Kleber and others (1981) showed that more than 80 percent of the children in a study failed to brush the lingual surfaces of the mandibular or maxillary teeth. Overall, 38 percent of the dental surfaces were not brushed. MacGreggor and Rugg-Gunn (1979) have similarly observed that the anterior labial surfaces were brushed most often and the lingual surfaces least often.

Findings for adults are no different. In 1946, Robinson found that toothbrushing was almost entirely confined to labial surfaces. More recently, Cumming and Löe (1973) found that labial surfaces had less plaque than lingual surfaces. Dexterity, even in adults, may be a factor. Kenney and others (1976) determined that manual dexterity of the preferred hand showed significant correlation with oral hygiene scores.

Observations of patient self-care are useful in designing an instructional program for each patient. Subsequent use of disclosing tablets after cleaning serves to reinforce the idea that inefficient or ineffective cleaning of certain surfaces results in the accumulation of plaque. To improve any physical skill, feedback must be provided. Feedback about performance may occur from a number of sources. Visual examination, disclosing solution, and self-inspection manuals can facilitate the feedback process (Baab and Weinstein, 1983). Patients must learn how to identify the problems in their own mouths.

EASILY ATTAINABLE GOALS. Once patient skill levels are identified, realistic and easily attainable goals or targets should be established. The tendency to go too far, too fast, should be avoided. The behavioral approach proceeds slowly, step by step, with considerable encouragement for the accomplishment of each step.

With patients whose skill levels are very low, or for whom cleaning is difficult because of broken down teeth, overhangs, and advanced periodontitis, we focus on the thorough cleaning of only a few teeth, usually the anterior teeth that are to be repaired or have just received curettage. On the subsequent appointment, give patients detailed feedback and encouragement. Then focus on additional teeth. This incremental approach works well with patients who have regular but ineffective home care habits. As a general rule, no patient should be given more than one cleaning aid until the previous one is mastered. Toothbrushes should proceed toothpicks, perio aids and proxibrushes, in our opinion. Dental floss, because it is so difficult to use well, should be reserved for the "advanced" patient.

We recommend disclosing the fearful patitent's teeth at every visit—not to criticize but to aid the patient in seeing plaque and evaluating his or her progress. This allows us to function as a coach. We watch our "athletes" perform and then give feedback designed to improve their skills. Praise and encouragement of the patient's efforts are crucial.

We also recommend brushing without toothpaste. This allows patients to see the teeth and evaluate their gums. Toothpaste makes it difficult to see bleeding resulting from unresolved gingivitis.

FACILITATE TRANSFER OF NEW SKILLS. Though patients may desire to alter their behaviors, old habits often interfere. As a general principle, learning to make new responses to old stimuli produces "negative transfer"; that is, the intrusion of old automatic habits into new behaviors should be expected. To facilitate transfer of this skill, we try to help patients make their oral care a self-conscious activity. Looking into a well-lighted mirror when cleaning may be of assistance to the patient because patients are taught new skills in the office using a mirror. Reminders are useful, such as monitoring charts and notes placed on mirrors or where oral self-care occurs. A copy of a chart we find useful is found in Figure 5-1. These charts are also useful in helping to establish realistic goals and objectives and provide considerable feedback. All of these instructions tend to alter not so much the responses but the stimuli or cues—the goal is to help the patients to perceive differences between the old habits and the new learning.

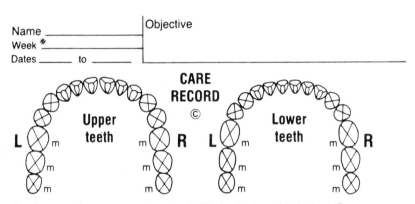

FIGURE 5-1. Patient Self-Care Help Chart.

CONCLUSION

This chapter is about practice management: in examining, planning and presenting care to fearful dental patients. It discusses scheduling, financing, emergencies, and preventive care. Some key points are:

1. Present a positive prognosis—avoid the "bad news" syndrome.

2. Listen to and work with the patient—respect their fears and preferences.

3. Adapt your procedures—be flexible—in planning, phasing, scheduling, and financing care.

Remember, for most fearful patients the biggest step is coming in for an examination. Respect this achievement and help them make this decision to seek treatment the basis for a long-standing relationship. Be in too big a hurry or push to hard for your views and they will not return.

QUESTIONS AND EXERCISES

1. List several strategies described in this chapter that will facilitate your examination and case presentation to a fearful patient.

2. List your objectives, as you would present them to a fearful patient, for an initial examination.

3. A fearful patient presents in your office with several endodontically involved molars and premolars. The patient has been in pain for several days and has hardly eaten or slept. Outline your strategy.

4. List several strategies for reducing cancellations by fearful patients.

5. Consider your current approach to home care instruction. What differences are there between what you do now and the approach suggested? How do you select whom you will work with? How do you set attainable goals?

SIX

Treatment of the Patient Who Fears Specific Procedures

There is considerable evidence (Mathews, 1978) that the most effective treatment of a wide variety of common fears involves the controlled exposure of patients to the phobic stimulus. The changes that occur in these situations are believed to involve not only conditioning but also an alteration in the patient's expectations (Lick and Bootzin, 1975; Kazdin and Wilcoxon, 1976; Bandera, 1977). Recall from Chapter 2 that a conditioned response is one that occurs automatically at the presentation of the stimulus. Graduated, controlled exposure therefore is the guiding principle behind the treatment of our patients who indicate fear of a specific dental procedure. Simply put, these patients are slowly but progressively exposed to the fearful procedure in a way that the expected negative experience (conditioned emotional response) does not occur. After repeated positive experiences, expectations of pain lessen and fear-related behaviors go away.

Providing the patient with some control is essential in preparing a fearful patient who is afraid of specific aversive procedures such as injections, rubber dams, or root canals. You will recall from Chapter 2 that researchers (see Averill, 1973; Thompson, 1981; and Miller, 1979) have defined four categories of control that may be helpful to the clinician in working with fearful patients. The first category is *information*. Most fearful patients like to know what sensations will be forthcoming. For example, we tell our patients that they will feel "pressure" during injections. Moreover, it is useful to provide information that includes both what the patient can expect, *and* what he or she can do about it when it occurs: "Sometimes patients experience difficulty breathing during an impression; it's better if you concentrate on breathing through your nose. . . ." There is vast psychological literature indicating that aversive events are much less stressful when they are predictable (Lazarus, 1966; Elliot, 1969; Seligman et al., 1971). Overall, specific information and explanation are useful for fearful patients.

The second type of control is *cognitive*. This has to do with how the patients think and feel about the situation they are in—the "meaning" of the event. Patients may believe they cannot control what they think about events. In such situations they may anticipate many negative events, which become self-fulfilling prophecies. Cognitive strategies such as distraction and hypnosis work best with these patients. This will be discussed in Chapter 8.

A third strategy involves enhancing *behavioral control*. Here the patient is provided with the opportunity to influence what is actually going on. For example, "Raise your hand when you're ready for us to start."

A fourth strategy is *retrospective control*. This is essentially *post-hoc* explanation. While a procedure may be aversive, for example tightening an orthodontic ligature, afterwards the dentist explains that the pain felt is a protective mechanism so he knows not to tighten the wire any further. Such an explanation may serve to lessen anticipation of subsequent appointments.

In this chapter we discuss the two types of control that are most useful for this type of fear: informational and behavioral control. Informational control involves explanation, behavioral control primarily signal mechanisms. These control mechanisms give the fearful individual a way to cope with the stress of a dental procedure. In Appendix C, the *Treatment Modality Checklist* summarizes the strategies we recommend for each type of patient.

INFORMATIONAL CONTROL

Mind-Body-Pain Model

Fearful people often act as if their behaviors are uncontrollable. Thus, we begin by explaining that pain tolerance is mediated by the attitudes, feeling, and attention focused on the event itself. We assert that the tension from inappropriate fight-flight responses increases sensitivity to pain. The arousal *itself* is aversive (Bolles and Fangslow, 1980). Thus, patients contribute to their own discomfort. Recall from Chapter 4 that these patients are afraid they will be unable to tolerate what they perceive will be excruciating pain.

We tell patients that when they are upset they are actually more likely to feel pain—real physical pain (Sternbach, 1968). Therefore, their job is to control their own emotions while our job is to assist them and to make the actual sensations as minimal as possible.

To demonstrate this principle clinically have the patient clench one hand while leaving the other relaxed. Pinch both hands between the thumb and first finger. The results will be that the "relaxed" condition results in less pain.

Preparation

Preparation and delivery of information to patients who are about to undergo a stressful procedure is extremely important. Do not surprise a patient. After a patient defines a procedure as stressful, the key issues are:

1. What and how much to tell the patient

2. When to tell them

3. How to tell them

There are three aspects of how much and what to tell the patient. First is information about technique. Generally, dentists tell patients too much about technical dental procedures and too little about things dealing with their safety and comfort. Technique should be concisely described in lay terms. "In the root canal treatment I carefully remove decay and infection that has involved the roots of the teeth." "When I do a filling in this tooth I will mainly be removing the old silver." The second concern is safety. Immediately prior to the event patients should be told what to expect. This should be accomplished so they know how to cooperate, and what measures are being taken for their safety. "The rubber dam is placed so you won't swallow any of the debris or dental materials while I'm working." "Your tongue is protected with the dam in place." The third aspect is suggestion for comfort. Tell patients that some procedures are done for their comfort. Also tell them how to respond if they are uncomfortable. "The topical anesthetic ointment will make your gums more comfortable while I clean this area. Please tell me if you want me to use it any-where else."

When should information be provided? Basic information outlining general strategies is appropriate during case presentations. Complex explanations, such as detailing each step of a procedure, or describing the feeling of a forceps extraction, should never be given far in advance of treatment unless requested. Misunderstandings at that point will lead to greater anticipation and apprehensiveness. It is more important to provide the information just before the stressful procedure. How you give information is the third key issue in preparing the patient. When telling a patient about a dental procedure, use all the senses. It is important to describe what the procedure may smell and feel like, what the instruments may sound like, and what the patient may see in the reflection in the dentist's safety glasses. Be very concerned about the words which are employed.

Take care in requests to the chairside assistant. Patients often interpret what the dentist says literally. An "enamel hatchet" may be a large object more appropriate to the woods or battlefield than to their mouths. Euphemisms are not difficult to find. Patients who fear specific procedures often have had no recent experience with the procedure. They have avoided for so long that the "avoidance" gradient is easily lowered with a few successful experiences, allowing them to approach the feared procedure in the future. Describing your procedure as "different" from the past is useful. We often use the analogy between propeller airplanes and commercial jets of the present, or the differences between the engine of an old '57 Chevy and a Datsun 280Z. We stress to the patient that dental procedures are now improved, that we are concerned about their experience, and that they have new coping skills they can apply to successfully tolerate the experience. Support and encouragement, with information, work especially well if the patient has not been in for treatment since childhood.

Tell-Show-Do

This procedure, so successful in children, is appropriate for adults. Such a procedure teaches patients "new" sensations.

Dentist: The first part of the cleaning procedure involves using an instrument to feel the surfaces of your teeth. Let me *show* you what I will do on this model (demonstrate). Perhaps you could hold the mirror and watch while I feel one of your teeth just as I did on the model? Can you feel the rough spot that my instrument is touching? It's tartar, or calculus, and is what causes tooth decay.

Patient: Yes it feels very big.

Dentist: Yes it does, it comes off easily (demonstration). When your gums heal they will be more comfortable. I will be feeling around each of the teeth very carefully to check for rough areas on your tooth. Then, I'll be cleaning them to make them smooth. When I'm doing this, it may sound a little strange and you will feel the instrument rubbing on your tooth but it will not be uncomfortable.

Another situation where *tell-show-do* works involves the high speed drill. The major problems with drilling are noise, vibration, and water. We explain the noise of the drill and water and the high speed vacuum as a cacophony. We ask them to experience this "music" before we begin. And at this point we demonstrate the noises and everything spinning around outside of the mouth. This eliminates surprise.

It is useful to keep the patient apprised of about how long the procedure will take and how far you have progressed. This kind of information keeps the patient in touch with reality. Time information helps keep you on schedule and reduces patient anxiety.

It's also helpful to ask several times during the appointment whether or not they would like to look at the work being done. It appears that patient willingness to look at work in progress is a sign fear is abating.

Another aspect of watching in the mirror is the ability of some patients to dissociate their fear from what they are observing. From the patient's perspective, it is as if the work is being performed on another person. Emotional responses that interfere with treatment may thus be minimized. The mirror is a handy tool.

BEHAVIORAL CONTROL

An analogy introducing the importance of control to patients involves removing a splinter. Most of us can use a needle to remove a splinter from our finger. While it is uncomfortable, few would describe it as unbearable or intensely painful. The reason it is bearable is because *we* control the needle and the importance attributed to it. The discomfort of a dental procedure is no worse, only the *control* aspect is different. Always frame explanations in terms patients can understand. An explanation to a religious person, a businessman, or a hippie would be different, as a metaphor meaningful to one may not be meaningful to another.

Signaling

Many patients fear not being able to control what the dentist is doing. Our view is that simply telling a patient he may signal that something hurts is not enough. For the fearful patient, active training by the dentist to instill and reinforce control is required. Signals as a control mechanism have positive implications for the success of treatment. When a patient accepts responsibility for indicating to the dentist his status, he will have overcome much of his helplessness. The patient's perception of control is critical.

Patients are not accustomed to participating in treatment. We find that encouraging the patient to watch procedures is helpful. It makes them more aware of what's going on and increases their control. Remember to allow the patient to keep his eye glasses on, and to use the patient mirror. Even if they decline, they know the opportunity is available.

Signal mechanisms are especially helpful to the patient with a rubber dam in place; simple hand or finger signals, a button connected to some kind of light or noisemaker, and a pad of paper and a pencil are useful. Initially there may be many patient interruptions. They are positive. For example in this scenario:

Patient: (Raises the hand)

Dentist: Are you having some discomfort?

182

Patient: (writes on pad) I need to go to the bathroom.

Dentist: I'm glad you told me. We have a stopping place just ahead and then you should be able to go. Is that OK?

Patient: Yes. Thank you.

Some patients will interrupt treatment frequently during the first several visits. It is critical that you do not show impatience at these interruptions. As patients become more comfortable and eager for treatment to proceed, they will interrupt less often. Realizing that "the dentist won't get mad at me" reduces the patient's feeling of anxiety and guilt.

Signaling Readiness to Proceed

As useful as signaling is for stopping treatment in case of pain or need for a break, we find that there is even a more effective strategy using signaling. Using it as a method to indicate a readiness to *proceed* is a more positive aspect of encouraging control. In this example we ask the patients to tell us when they are ready for an injection.

Dentist: I'm going to be using this fruit flavored topical ointment to make your skin numb around this tooth. (Pointing) I'm going to smear some of the ointment on the skin above the tooth, and I'd like you to let me know when you can feel the numbness or tingling or cold or warm feeling that the topical anesthetic provides. That's the time when we'll know that that area is numb."

Patient: (after a few minutes) Yes, now I think I can feel the numbness beginning.

Dentist: Good, then let's move on to the next step.

Few, if any patients, will fail to respond to these suggestions. Be sure to reinforce the patient for being ready to proceed. If they do fail, it is a sign to rethink your diagnosis of the problem.

Failing to Respond to Signals

Many patients complain that the dentist does not respond to signals—verbal or otherwise. If you have instructed a patient to give a signal for needing a rest break, you must honor your commitment. Remember that with the fearful patient, control is paramount. Not living up to your end of this implied social contract reduces patient trust.

The dentist needs to remember that relinquishing control of these aspects of treatment is technically unimportant. Flexibility in rest breaks or duration of treatment will allow the patient control.

Behavioral Strategies Useful with the Injection

It's ironic that the procedure that allows patients to be treated virtually free of pain is the one that they often fear the most. Many are afraid of the pain of the injection; others exaggerate the extent of the needle penetration. We'll discuss these basic problems here. Other aspects of the use of anesthetics and reactions to anesthetics are in Chapter 3.

It often is helpful to begin exposure to anesthetic injection using an infiltration rather than a block. We do this because the results are very predictable and pain of injection is minimal with careful technique. However, similar procedures can be followed for injections in any area. We are not reluctant to give injections in any part of the mouth at the initial treatment visit, if that is what is needed. This includes palatal injections and other injections that may be perceived by the dentist as painful. The following scenario describes how we prepare our patients through information and behavioral control.

Patient: I'm really concerned about the injection.

Dentist: I understand your concern. The source of discomfort with injections is the pressure. The needle puncture itself lasts only a second and generally patients don't even feel it because we use topical anesthetic on the skin. If I go very slowly, you will find that the pressure created by the anesthetic in the tissue is not painful. However, you will always feel the pressure. That's good

HERMAN®

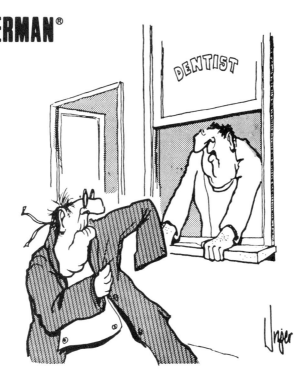

"What happened! Did I touch a nerve?"

because it will remind you of the anesthetic working. I'd like you to imagine first of all that your hand or your foot has gone to sleep. I think you can probably remember what that feels like can't you?

Patient: Yes.

Dentist: Imagine that it's gone to sleep and that it feels very heavy and numb but it doesn't hurt. Can you feel that?

Patient: Yes, I can feel that.

Dentist: OK, I would like to put some topical anesthetic ointment on your tongue to see if you can feel a numbness in your tongue.

185

Patient: (after 15 seconds) Yes, I have the feeling in my tongue.

Dentist: OK, that's very good. Now I'd like to put some of the topical ointment on your gums. Sometimes it's harder for patients to be able to feel it here, but I'd like you to try and see if you can feel it. Even if you can't feel it, you know that the same feeling of numbness is going to exist in the skin. I'll paint some on now and you take just a moment and tell me if and when you can feel the anesthetic.

Patient: (After 30 seconds) Yes, I can feel the numbness now.

Dentist: Very good. It's difficult for some patients to feel this. It's good that you're able to do it. Now, I'm going to lift your lip and administer some additional anesthetic. The skin is very numb. You will experience some pressure, which won't be painful. And as you feel that pressure, you will feel the spreading of the numbness.

Dentist: I'm going very slowly. I'm about half done now (about 15–20 seconds). The slower I go, the more comfortable it is for you. I'm three-quarters done. Now I'm done. You look like you're feeling very comfortable.

Patient: Yes I didn't feel the needle at all.

Dentist: But you did feel the pressure, didn't you.

Patient: Yes I felt the pressure. And I can feel this numbness spreading.

Note that good technique is required. Needles should be placed carefully and the anesthetic administered slowly. Thirty seconds or more is required to empty a 1.8-ml carpule. Pressure anesthesia or additional topical anesthetic should always be used wherever the dentist or hygienist anticipates there may be discomfort. Our reading of the situation is that the key variables are preparation (using the topical as above) and care in injecting slowly. In our view, other factors such as anesthetic temperature or needle gauge are relatively unimportant.

One additional word about needles. One advantage of beginning with an infiltration in the anterior is the short needle. Usually after that first good experience with an anesthetic, we try to show the syringe to the patient. At this time we show them that little of the needle actually penetrates the skin and explain that the long needle is for safety. With this example patients will generalize and then anticipate, even if the injection is a mandibular block, that the needle does not penetrate very far. This will aid them in being more comfortable with the injection procedure.

Case Example: Substituting Behaviors for Patient Fear of Injection During Graduated Exposure

We recently treated a patient whose story allows us to demonstrate how to put these strategies together. This patient had a long history of intense fear of medical and dental injections. She resisted injections by biting the dentist, grabbing the syringe, or bolting from the chair. Her last visit to the dentist was two years ago. This was the only dental procedure she was afraid of. She was a competent person who ran her own business and managed many personal problems. She took care of sick relatives as well as her own work and family. Paradoxically, sewing machine needles, which routinely caused her injury in her business, did not upset her at all. She had no other fears and tolerated scaling and drilling of a non-vital tooth without anesthetic quite well during the initial three appointments. No problems occurred and we got to know her well.

After the initial visits she agreed to try to solve the anesthetic problem. The steps in desensitizing this patient were:

1. Presentation of the mind-body-pain model
2. Tell-show-do
3. Substituting a coping for a panic response.

Let's focus on the third part because it is the key to success. Two one-half hour appointments were required.

The approach for this problem involved rehearsals of the desired behaviors. For diagnostic purpose, at the first appointment we told the patient we would rehearse by bringing the syringe to her mouth (with the cover on the needle). Everything went fine as the topical was placed but when the syringe came near, the circumoral muscles tensed. After this, heart rate increased and the patient reported being panicky.

The patient was asked to rest for a few minutes and then indicate when we could try a second rehearsal. This time we asked the patient to practice tensing the masseter, clenching, and then to sigh deeply. When sighing, the masseter relaxed. So when the lip was retracted and the syringe placed this time (again with the cover in place), the dentist commanded the patient to sigh at the first sign of muscle tension. The patient still tensed the muscles a little but did not reach for the syringe, turn away, or show any of the previous interfering behaviors. The patient was praised for her effort. After resting, the clenching-relaxing behavior was practiced again, when the patient indicated she was ready.

The analogy used in explaining the need for this practice was as follows: "We want your desired reaction to be automatic, just like putting on the car brakes when you see a red traffic light. The more you practice relaxing (or driving), the more automatic it becomes when you are aware that you are getting upset." In this way, the patient gains control over the procedure.

On the third try, the patient successfully allowed the trial to proceed without any resistance, all the while breathing deeply. Again she was praised for her success. At the conclusion of the appointment she was given homework to practice imagining the syringe and using the clenching-relaxing exercise. This was to be done regularly before the second appointment.

At the second appointment, after another rehearsal, the injection was administered successfully. In less than one hour, a seemingly insurmountable problem was solved and the patient went on to be a highly cooperative and satisfactory participant in dental care. The key element was behavioral control.

Breathing: a Behavioral Technique to Induce Bodily Relaxation

Westerners have only recently become aware of the importance of breathing habits in the role of relaxation. Relaxed patients simply do not feel nearly as much discomfort as those who are tense (Thompson, 1977). Thus, it is a good idea to employ some simple techniques that will enhance relaxation. For centuries, breathing exercises have been an integral part of mental, physical, and spiritual development in the Orient and India. As the West hurries to catch up with the East in understanding and utilizing proper breath control, it has borrowed heavily from the teachings of Yoga. The underlying goal of all Yoga is to enable a person through self-discipline to control his or her body and mind.

When an insufficient amount of fresh air reaches someone's lungs, blood is not properly oxygenated. Poorly oxygenated blood contributes to anxiety states, depression, and fatigue and makes stressful situations such as dental treatment harder to cope with (Spreads, 1978).

One technique begins by asking the patients to fill the lungs and then to "sigh" or exhale slowly. Your personal demonstration of this simple technique is useful. Remind the patient that the muscles are much more relaxed when exhaling. Physically guide the patient through four or five very slow breaths and request that he or she continue for at least ten minutes. Most anxious patients will be more comfortable, and you can proceed as soon as patient breathing becomes slow and regular. This exercise is useful for most fearful patients and especially recommended for patients who are afraid of specific stimuli such as the injection. Another technique involves focusing on exhalation. Begin by asking the patient to complete two slow and deep breathing cycles, as described above. Then instruct the patient to breathe out and not to inhale for as long as possible. When breathing can no longer be restrained, tell him to inhale and to attend to the relief experienced. Follow this respiratory relief by two slow and deep breathing cycles (Longo, 1984). Repeat for as long as needed. Many fearful patients tend to hold their breath during dental procedures. An alert chairside assistant can help patients pace their breathing. The assistant might lightly press on the patient's shoulder to remind them to exhale. You can use similar procedures to pace the breathing of a patient who is likely to hyperventilate. This procedure will be helpful to patients in a variety of tense situations, especially during injections, or after initial placement of the rubber dam.

Try using breathing before and during impressions. Practice the procedure with an empty tray. Time the practice so the patient learns how long the real impression procedure will last. When the patient indicates it's OK to begin, do the procedure in the same way it was rehearsed. Some anxious behavior may still result. Nonetheless, praise the patient for successful coping, and then let him regain his composure before proceeding. Successive successful experiences will result in desensitization to this procedure.

Dentists and auxiliaries will want to practice these techniques themselves. Proper breathing is an antidote to stress for staff as well as for patients.

ENHANCING POST-TREATMENT COMFORT

Dental treatment and the recovery interval are periods of psychological and physical stress for patients. The physical stress comes from the actual tissue damage. The psychological stress can occur because of the patient's expectations of being harmed during treatment, or of experiencing complications following it. It is clear that the degree of physical trauma affects post-operative recovery. However, it has only been recently recognized that psychological factors influence actual physical aspects of post-surgical recovery.

Research by George et al. (1980) shows a correlation between healing rate after surgery, the patient's acceptance of his or her condition, and the *meaning* of the event to the individual. Patients who attached a positive meaning to their situation healed more quickly, perceived their problems as surmountable, and saw their condition as a temporary setback. It was found that oral surgery patients who had expectations of post-surgical pain had more reported pain and slower healing that those patients with high expectations of a rapid recovery.

These and other studies indicate that attitude affects not only the actual physiological rate of recovery, but influences the patient's self-reports of pain and post-operative complications, i.e., repeat visits and 2:00 AM emergency calls.

Our clinical experience with patients at the Dental Fears Research Clinic illustrates the importance of psychological factors in post-operative recovery. The fearful patient is far more likely to experience difficulties both during and following the appointment than is a non-anxious patient. Those patients with Generalized Anxiety (see Chapter 8) are the most likely to call following restorative work with questions or complaints of pain. This may be because of their characteristic tendency to worry. We employ two basic strategies to enhance recovery and decrease post-operative complications. The first technique focuses on what can be termed suggestion in the broad sense of the word. The second focuses on cognitive coping techniques that we teach to help the patient deal with the procedure itself as well as the recovery period.

Suggestion and the Role of Information

Much has been written about how much information should be given prior to and following surgical procedures. Clum (1979) indicated that those patients who received additional information experienced more post-operative pain than those who were treated as usual. Other studies tend to confirm that simply giving more information is not effective in preparing the patient for surgery and, with some patients, may be counterproductive. This is not to say we should avoid providing the patient information, but it points to the fact that it is not sufficient in helping the patient cope optimally with restorative procedures. Research by Schmitt (1973) and George (1980) indicates that working to modify the patient's expectations and attitudes towards the event results in fewer post-operative complications and a more rapid recovery.

As we mentioned previously in this chapter, we attempt to begin dental treatment with procedures that are less threatening to the patient in order to desensitize him to the dental environment. This allows us to spend time talking with the patient preparing for the more fearful procedure. This *includes* providing information, but it is used in the context of helping the patient enhance positive expectations towards the event.

It should be remembered that information is a form of "suggestion." Thus, it is important that all communication with the patient be geared towards improving the patient's recovery. A sense of control may be important. For example, suggestions that there are positive actions that the patient can take to speed recovery, such as warm salt water rinses, may help provide the patient with a sense of control over recovery. Reassurance that help is available, if needed, also seems to improve the patient's acceptance of condition and mitigates the individual's tendency to worry.

We attempt to help the patient place future appointments in a positive perspective. We find that for many patients successfully being able to complete work they have long feared and avoided is symbolic of "getting their act together" and is perceived as a significant accomplishment. At every step, we provide positive reinforcement for their progress and encourage their efforts to overcome their fears. Immediately prior to the procedure we rehearse with the patient the coping techniques to be used, and briefly reexplain what it is that we are going to do during the actual procedure, the rationale behind it, and what we expect will happen immediately following recovery. We provide the most detailed information, not about treatment procedures, but about what to expect during the post-operative period. We try to identify both sensations that are part of the normal recovery and sensations that are abnormal.

The evening following restorative treatment, we routinely call those patients we feel have a high probability of experiencing post-operative difficulties. This includes all patients described in Chapter 9 and most distrustful individuals (Chapter 7). This technique allows us to contact the patient at *our* convenience and eliminate most late-night calls at home—and reinforces our efforts at maintaining rapport.

Additionally, we have created a series of short handouts which we give out following each restorative appointment. They explain in writing the points that we have discussed verbally.

Coping Strategies

The second major strategy involves teaching the patient cognitive coping techniques. Numerous studies indicate that these are effective in reducing post-operative complications. In a study of 97 abdominal surgery patients,

Egbert (1964) found recovery was improved through teaching presurgical patients physical and psychological coping techniques. Following surgery they rated their pain as less intense, requested less medication, and were discharged earlier. In a study of 25 male patients scheduled for general surgery procedures, Schmitt and Wooldridge (1973) found that the patient group who met with a nurse prior to surgery to discuss their fears and concerns reported less post-operative pain and was discharged earlier than a comparable control group. Finally, Langer et al. (1974) found in a study of 60 patients undergoing general surgery that giving patients a coping device for dealing with post-surgical pain (directing attention to the favorable consequences of their recent surgery) reduced pain reports significantly more than information alone.

A simple coping technique that is useful during the post-operative recovery period is self-distraction. The patient is encouraged to resume normal activities as soon as possible and to read, watch TV, etc. during rest periods rather than lying about focusing on pain. Also, we tell patients, prior to extraction, to prepare for a special, relaxing, low-key evening. Another pragmatic technique is the use of mental and muscle relaxation instructions, which are useful in helping patients cope with immediate stress in the operatory as well as during the post-surgical period.

CONCLUSION

This chapter was about the fearful patient who is afraid of a specific procedure. For aversive stimuli such as injections or impressions, we suggest graduated exposure with explanation and behavioral control strategies. Roles for the dentist, hygienist, and assistant are recommended. Key clinical techniques suggested in this chapter are:

1. Patient preparation and information
2. Signalling
3. Substituting coping responses such as breathing exercises
4. Rehearsals

193

Finally, suggestions are given on how to enhance post-operative comfort.

QUESTIONS AND EXERCISES

1. Describe at least one way in which you can facilitate your patient's sense of control from each of the four categories: Information, Cognitive, Behavioral, Retrospective.

2. Discuss the concept of perceived control over the treatment procedures with one of your next patients. Ask, using your own words, how much control they feel they actually have. That is, what do you think they can or cannot do? How would you classify it? Ask if they would like more or less control. Why or why not?

3. Try to explain the mind-body-pain model to a patient. Does it make sense to them? What examples do you use to explain the concept?

4. What does research indicate as the post-operative preparation or information that is most useful in helping patients cope during the recovery period?

SEVEN

Treatment of the Distrustful Patient

GENERAL CONSIDERATIONS

As indicated in Chapters 2 and 6, both research and clinical experience show that fearful behaviors in the operatory often originate in a perceived lack of control over the dentist, dental hygienist, and assistant. At the extreme, some patients feel that in going to the dentist they give up all control. They may believe they cannot influence the dentist to stop a procedure or rest, even for a moment. When an aversive experience occurs (i.e., "the dentist hurt me"), the feeling of helplessness accentuates the anxiety the patient brought to the dental setting.

Distrust occurs when we fail to establish rapport, belittle fears or self-care habits, or otherwise fail to anticipate or respond to patient concerns. The distrustful patient may appear angry, want everything in writing, and may wish to have a friend or spouse in the operatory. He or she may want a mirror to watch every move you make and request a lot of information. This patient is alert and sensitive to your personal and professional demeanor and your assessment of him or her.

Distrust results in an unwillingness to delegate control to the dentist. As suggested in Chapter 2, distrust usually originates from direct experiences: "The dentist wouldn't stop when I told him it hurt to drill." Other common presenting complaints are, "The dentist is always in a rush, he doesn't know me as a person" or "I wanted to have my teeth cleaned in two short appointments and the dentist said I was being silly." On the other hand, distrust can originate indirectly: "My friend told me root canals are incredibly painful." Or, distrust may stem in part from nondental experiences such as difficult medical procedures or poor rapport with physicians that generalizes to dentists.

BEHAVIORAL CONTROL

Recall from Chapter 2 that researchers have defined four categories of control helpful to the clinician in working with fearful patients: information, cognitive, retrospective, and behavioral. The best strategy for treating dental fear based on distrust is enhancing behavioral control. This, as with all successful therapy, must be done within a trusting relationship. So in this chapter we will try to explain how to build a trust relationship with a fearful person and then go on to suggest how to enhance the patient perceived control. However, it should be recognized that this approach is useful in treating other forms of dental fear as well. Nonetheless, in the treatment of fear based on distrust it is fundamental.

In Chapter 6 we discussed patients who were afraid they would not tolerate specific procedures. Loss of control of themselves was an intolerable situation. However, the fear of loss of control can manifest itself in other ways. Anger and distrust result when the fear is turned *outward* and the patient places the blame or the cause of the fear on the health professional. While we often have no objective way of assessing these prior experiences, once pinpointed, the problem of control can be used to our advantage in treating the *fear* as well as the dental problem. Because this anxious patient is distrustful, he or she needs active demonstrations of his or her participatory role in treatment. Many dentists fear the patient will make requests that interfere with treatment. Examples of these are: "I don't wish to have anesthetic," or "I won't let you take that impression, it makes me gag."

Treatment of distrustful patients requires enhancement of their sense of personal control. Reassurance, "Everything will be all right—just trust me," especially when there is little personal rapport, will have a negative effect and only reinforce patients' prior distrust. In Appendix C the *Treatment Modality Checklist* summarizes the strategies we recommend for these patients.

BUILDING A TRUSTING RELATIONSHIP

We will now discuss the key elements of building a trusting relationship. They are: rapport building, two-way communication, patient initiated control and decision making, and dentist-initiated time structuring.

Rapport Building

Some patients constantly interrupt what we're doing wanting to know every detail of procedures before we do them, no matter how trivial.

Others are suspicious, waiting for us to trick or hurt them. Of the four major diagnostic categories of fearful patients, distrustful individuals are most likely to respond positively to information and explanations. They like things "out in the open" and often appreciate hearing the "scientific rationale" behind each procedure as it is performed.

Rapport must be established with this patient *early*. We believe fearful patients form impressions of the dentist in the first few minutes of an initial encounter. Thus, the first three to five minutes of this appointment should be spent trying to learn about the patient. A common complaint of patients referred to the Dental Fears Research Clinic at the University of Washington is that the "dentist didn't know me as a person." Most of this time should be spent listening to concerns and exploring patient interests. Rapport is a harmonious relationship; the goal is to make the patient comfortable while getting acquainted. This does not legitimize continual "small talk" about the weather, current events, the local sports team, and so on. Rapport is likely to be encouraged when you discuss the patient's problems early on and demonstrate real interest in the patient's life. The ability to ask a question that requires more than a yes/no answer and just listen is extremely important here. Make notations on the patient's chart about his or her concerns and special interests. Refer to them each time you meet with the patient. Rapport with a distrustful patient must be renewed and reinforced at each visit. It cannot be taken for granted and must be an important consideration at *each* appointment. This is a unique consideration in working with distrust.

Our experience suggests that the competent yet caring professional is best for the distrusting patient. What does this mean? First, be prepared and ready to treat this patient. Be on time. One patient we recently treated complained that the dentist did not have her insurance predetermination in hand when he discussed her care plan. Do not interrupt the patient or take a condescending tone. Patients who feel vulnerable are often acutely sensitive to discourtesies. Second, examine your environment. What is on the walls, the music, etc. What does it project? Your reception area gives patients an impression of the sort of relationship they will have with you. Try to warm up the environment. Decorations and expensive artwork are not necessary. A few pictures of your family or of you holding a string of fish, or your child's artwork can give even the most angry patient an image of the dentist as a real person. Greet the patient outside the operatory. These are important sources of non-verbal communication.

Third, remember to make eye contact and be sensitive to your posture. Demonstrate your concern by your non-verbal gestures. Touching the patient gently with permission is much better than just verbal reassurance. Do not hurry. Hurrying, which is a major patient complaint about dentistry, conveys to the patient that you are not interested in him or her. Lean intently toward the patient when you are trying to show interest in what he is saying.

With such patients it is very easy to forget that the general opinion of patients about dentists is very positive. It is important not to take personally the indication of distrust from an anxious person. Try, instead, to ask the patient how you can act to facilitate his care, to improve the experience. Establish *positive* expectations. Let the patient know you feel comfortable with his problem and want to hear his thoughts, feelings, and reactions so you will be able to work with him to have a good experience. Such an encounter might sound like this:

Patient: I'm afraid to let you look at my gums because the last dentist really made me feel guilty for letting them get this bad.

Dentist: I understand. After I look at your gums, I will try to give you a full explanation of the situation and recommendations you can think about. You can ask questions, then you can decide what you want to do.

A final element of the rapport building process is the modeling of openness. As we have just discussed, fearful patients are afraid of being put down. A positive statement by the dental assistant or hygienist that reveals something about herself is useful.

Dental Assistant: You know, I used to be anxious about going to the dentist.

Patient: Really?

Dental Assistant: I have always been uptight about sitting in the chair. But I found out that our dentist really tried to get to know me and understood my fears. Now I'm really comfortable.

Such statements allow the patient to be himself or herself and to express concerns about treatment without fear of embarrassment or belittlement. It is important to note (and easy to forget) that the behavior of the staff is very important in forging positive relationships with these patients. Most of the work in establishing rapport is routinely done by the staff in the office. Your staff may be very competent in this area.

Two Areas of Special Concern

Distrustful patients are especially embarrassed about being fearful and about the condition of their oral health and hygiene habits.

EMBARRASSMENT OVER BEING FEARFUL. Patients who are embarrassed about being fearful are afraid the dentist will not take their fears seriously. Such patients may say to you that they feel they are being childish. They know it's irrational, yet they feel uncomfortable being in the dentist's office. For example:

Patient: I know other people can stand it but I just can't take the sound of that scratching on my teeth when they're being cleaned. Can't you put me out or something?

Hygienist: I understand the scratching on your teeth is very uncomfortable for you. It's not that unusual. Many other patients are sensitive to this feeling. Let's try and figure out what we can do to minimize your discomfort. Perhaps we can try. . . .

An *inappropriate* response would be:

Hygienist: Our tooth cleaning procedures really don't hurt and I'm sure you can deal with it.

First, of course, the patient would not be in this state if he could deal with it. Second, the assumption that pain is the primary issue is probably incorrect because most tooth cleaning procedures do not hurt. Most apprehensive patients would interpret such a response as a "put-down." They are not willing to trust you just because you say it will not hurt. An empathetic response is a far better approach to this problem than a response that denies the legitimacy of the patient's feelings by premature reassurance. Stress your concern for the patient's needs. The best reassurance you can provide is that you will attempt to deal with the patient's perceived problems.

EMBARRASSMENT OVER ORAL CLEANLINESS. In our experience, many fearful patients have poor oral hygiene accentuated by lack of contact with dentistry. They are sensitive to criticism, however benign, and most dental professionals criticize. It is almost as if we would prefer that all our patients come to us healthy. It should not be so surprising that many anxious and fearful patients arrive with very poor oral hygiene. Imagine this scenario (our patients do):

Patient: I'm really embarrassed to let you look in my mouth. I haven't been taking very good care of my mouth. (Dental Hygienist looks into mouth.)

Hygienist: You're right, this is really a mess! Don't you care about keeping your teeth?

Perhaps a better approach would have been:

Hygienist: I can see you have an infection in your mouth. I'm glad you came to see us now because it's possible to cure it, especially if we have your active participation. Later on, with your permission, we would like to teach you some special cleaning skills that you can use in helping control the problem. It is difficult to reach some areas of your mouth. . . . Do you have any questions? . . . . If you should have a question later, please feel free to. . . .

It is important to remember that these patients will take any sign of belittlement as a confirmation that they should put off dental care. They

202

may rationalize avoidance by saying "this dental hygienist doesn't understand my problem" or "this dentist isn't willing to be accommodating." The dentist or hygienist who is successful with the anxious or fearful patient is *accepting* of the problem and *flexible* in its remediation.

Two-Way Communication

Two-way communication is essential to working with the distrustful patient. These patients need to learn that they can exercise some personal control in what they perceive as a dangerous situation. The vehicle is communication.

HERMAN®

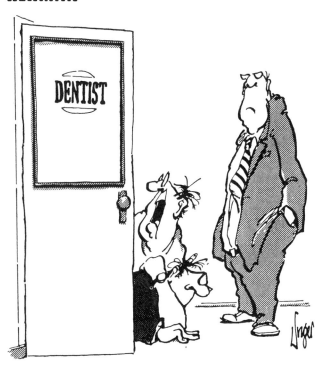

"Grab his legs!"

Not long ago this type of anxious patient would have spent a lot of time rinsing his or her mouth and spitting into the cuspidor. Patients will often use these types of maneuvers as a substitute for telling you what the problem is. As a clinician you need to tell the patient that he needs to let you know how he is doing. The distrustful patient feels like he cannot control what the dental professional will do. He feels powerless and like a victim. You might look at the solution to this as *assertiveness training* for the patient. Assertiveness is simply being able to communicate with dental personnel one's likes and dislikes and questions.

Another example of this phenomenon is the patient who continually asks: "Why is this treatment going to be better?" The best response is "Please tell me what you would like me to do to help treatment be a good experience for *you.*" You may also need to tell the patient which areas he should give you feedback about. These preferences are important to the success of treatment. For example, the nonassertive patient may not feel comfortable in telling the dentist that the anesthesia is not completely effective, that he gets dizzy when the chair is tipped all the way back, or she does not understand the treatment plan or the costs of treatment. Unasked questions add considerably to distrust.

Imagine how you would feel as a patient if you had to sit there and bear the discomfort and couldn't say anything. Wouldn't your apprehensiveness grow? Many patients will simply fail to report being hurt out of concern that the dentist may make light of their discomfort. A previous dentist may have said "Sit still, it will only be a little bit longer," or "It's not very uncomfortable. This isn't a very bad cavity." Try to reverse roles and imagine yourself as your patient under these circumstances.

Working with patients so that they can be comfortable in communicating their desires will reduce the frustration of uncompleted treatment plans and failed appointments associated with not knowing the patient's wishes. Perhaps some examples will be helpful.

Case Examples

The first patient is an older woman who has generally taken good care of her teeth but now finds herself in the position of having a failing lower fixed bridge. She is already partially edentulous in the lower arch. She visited a prosthodontist who strongly recommended reconstruction of the upper and lower teeth including fixed and removable appliances. She had her teeth cleaned by the dentist's hygienist and then reported to the office on three separate occasions to begin restorative treatment. *Each time she would not allow the dentist to begin.* Nevertheless, in none of the visits did she tell the dentist she was not prepared to go ahead with this extensive treatment. It simply did not meet her needs. Yet, she was not assertive enough (comfortable) in her communication with the dentist to be able to ask questions or to tell him that she didn't want to go ahead.

We recently received a letter about a second problem patient from a dentist who was puzzled and frustrated over losing a $4,000 case. The patient had expressed her fears initially, and the dentist recommended some specialty treatment prior to the crown and bridge. While the patient complied, she found the specialists impersonal and had questions about the cost. While the patient returned several times for consultations and agreed to begin the crown and bridge, she changed dentists before treatment could commence. Her assessment: she felt that she had no say at all in who provided treatment and began to "feel abused."

Patient-Initiated Control and Decision Making

TREATMENT PREFERENCES. As we discussed in Chapter 5, it is essential to work with patients to encourage their stating their views and preferences. Imagine this scenario:

Patient: Doctor, you know, I know that I have gum problems and these broken teeth in the front of my mouth.

Dentist: I see, do you have any preferences about which problem we work on first?

Patient: Yes, I'm extremely concerned about the way that my front teeth look.

Dentist: I'm glad you told me that because I think then I would like to recommend that we begin our treatment by trying to remove the
decay and to replace missing parts of this front tooth with a cosmetic filling.

Patient: I'm really excited about looking better. That sounds fine to me.

What's different about this approach? Most clinicians have been
trained to care for problems in priority order: emergent/acute problems,
disease control, and rehabilitation. Cosmetics are usually a lower priority,
in part because many of us believe patients will not return for posterior
restorations if the anteriors are done first. In our experience with the distrustful patient, failure to attend to their concerns will result in cancellations or "disappearance." We encourage you to do something that shows
early on. Repair anteriors, even if temporarily. Clean anteriors, remove
calculus, and stain. If you do this, the patient can experience some success,
feel good about what the dentist has done, and is much more likely to return.

SAFETY. Another distrustful patient reported feeling dizzy and unable to swallow when the chair was reclined. One of us suggested to the
patient that she tell her dentist so he could adjust the chair. With some encouragement, the patient asserted her feelings. When the dentist adjusted
the chair for her there was a palpable sigh of relief and triumph on her
face when she knew she had some control.

With this patient, we negotiated a solution to the chair position. We
agreed to gradually tilt the chair back progressively over a series of appointments. Each time we would record the chair position in the chart and
move it back only as far as the patient was comfortable. After a couple of
visits, the problem disappeared and we were back to the original reclined
position.

WATCHING THE DENTIST. The distrustful patient always carefully attends to what is going on. This attention may be focused and made
useful by furnishing the patient with a mirror. Watching the procedure

will allow the patient to know what is going on. It makes the treatment being received concrete and dispels inaccurate perceptions. The patient's desire to watch should be encouraged and viewed as part of the patient's participation in his or her oral health care.

APPOINTMENT SCHEDULING. Patients can express their preferences for the time of day, length of appointment, or intervals between appointments. It is important to allow some flexibility about such things. Imagine these two scenarios:

Receptionist: Doctor would like you to make an appointment now for preparing your tooth for a crown.

Patient: That's a stressful procedure for me and I would prefer to have it done in the middle of the day since my husband can come with me.

Receptionist: I'm sorry, Doctor only does these procedures in the morning.

Patient: Oh, I see.

Now the alternative.

Receptionist: Do you have any preferences about when your next appointment is? It will be for your crown.

Patient: Oh I'm relieved you told me that. I would really like to come in the middle of the day because my husband can drive me.

Receptionist: Good, I'm glad you told me that. Ordinarily, Doctor Gooddentist doesn't do these procedures in the middle of the day but I know that he's very eager to accommodate you. How about . . . ?

Another problem is the interval between visits. Some patients just want to get treatment over with and wish to come very often now that they have gotten up their courage to come in the first place. Others may wish to have rest breaks in between their appointments. Generally speaking, this timing is unimportant to the success of treatment, and flexibility is rewarded with fewer cancellations.

Time-structuring

Just knowing how long a procedure will last helps a patient cope; so do dentist-planned breaks. These short respites are important to avoid minor discomfort becoming unbearable. A positive example involves the endodontist to whom we sometimes refer.

The patient, a woman in her late forties, had had much previous treatment. She suffers from chronic back pain and has difficulty sitting in the chair comfortably for long periods. Her previous treatment experiences were traumatic, and she sought care from the Dental Fears Research Clinic after avoiding treatment for a defective bridge, several failed endodontic treatments, and at least one symptomatic, previously untreated tooth.

After a diagnostic session, our clinic staff felt that we could not treat the dental needs in a timely way, so a specialty referral was necessary. With the patient's consent, we arranged for the endodontist to see her that day. We gave him explicit instructions to structure the appointments with 5-minute periods of treatment followed by one-minute rest breaks out of the chair, and to give the patient control over the length of the rest breaks. With this simple strategy, the patient received care in a humane manner and gave us glowing reports of her treatment.

SELF-HELP STRATEGIES

The distrustful patient is a great candidate for non-judgmental home care instruction. Being able to control the disease process permits a measure of independence from health care providers these patients relish. It is a tremendous opportunity for the dentist or staff to praise the patient's progress and support his or her efforts. As with other care with this patient, a well-prepared professional is more effective. For example:

Hygienist: The bacteria that live on your teeth cause the redness and bleeding in your gums. I'd like to apply some food coloring on your teeth and stain these bacterial colonies so they are easier to see. (Demonstrate)

Patient: What do I look for?

Hygienist: See the red debris between your teeth?

Patient: Yes.

Hygienist: Good, this red stuff indicates the bacteria that you need to consistently remove in order to return your gums to health.

We suggest keeping records in the chart, such as a plaque map, and using these records each visit to reinforce progress. Set readily achievable goals and move forward one step at a time. This way you will be able to find something to praise at each appointment. Sincere social reinforcement helps dispel distrust. You may want to consult the part of Chapter 5 on home care instruction if you have not read this already.

SIGNIFICANT OTHER. Another way for patients to overcome lack of control is having another person in the operatory. A patient who is afraid of being hurt, or simply needs reassurance, may wish to bring a trusted relative or friend into the operatory. There's simply no reason not to allow it! In another setting Sousa and others reported in 1980 that in healthy Guatemalan women, a supportive lay woman, a "doula," had a positive effect on length of labor, rate of perinatal problems, and mother-infant interaction. This added social support may have a positive reassuring effect on dental patients as well.

At the University, we recently treated a young, intelligent woman who initially was angry and distrustful. She reported a series of unpleasant experiences previously with physicians and had not been to a dentist in more than 10 years. She requested that a friend be present in the operatory during the examination. Our staff acknowledged her concern and gave the friend the assistant's stool right at chairside. In retrospect, the friend was our biggest advocate and really encouraged our patient to get needed treatment. Having the "significant other" on hand was the kind of social reinforcement this patient needed.

CONCLUSION

This chapter is about dental fears stemming from distrust. We recommend serious efforts at rapport building, two-way communication, emphasis on patient decision making, and dentist time-structuring. Enhancing behavioral control is the key to success with the distrustful patient.

QUESTIONS AND EXERCISES

1. List several specific means by which you can facilitate gaining patients' trust. Write out specific questions and statements to begin this process. Practice these on your next patients.

2. Cite some specific ways in which dental auxiliaries can set the tone for an open, trusting relationship with patients.

3. Write two different scenarios that might occur with a new patient who seeks care at your office with a mouth that is in need of extensive restoration and home care. First write out the worst set of interactions you can think of, one in which the patient is made to feel very ashamed and embarrassed. Second, write out a conversation in which you attempt to project yourself as an interested, concerned person and health care provider.

EIGHT

Treatment of the Patient with Generalized Anxiety

GENERAL CONSIDERATIONS

As you will recall from Chapter 4, patients with generalized anxiety experience difficulty with all kinds of stressful situations. They internalize their fear by saying "I can't cope." They can not think of an effective way to gain control over the events that bother them and very often report being unable to alter how they think. Such patients may spend endless hours worrying about their future dental appointment. As the time nears, they lose sleep and report an inability to concentrate and a myriad of other anxiety symptoms.

We recently saw a patient in this diagnostic category who had successfully completed several prophylaxis visits. He arrived for an endodontic treatment visit looking tired, drawn, and emotionally drained.

Receptionist: We're really glad you were able to come in today. This visit is important for your care.

Patient: I was up all night. I couldn't sleep. I feel really silly. If I had more self-discipline I'd do better.

Receptionist: We know you'll be using the skills you have learned.

Patient: I'll try but I don't think I can do it. I feel so childish.

It follows, then, that successful treatment of this patient involves changing what he thinks he can master. We try to shift his attention from "just waiting for the dentist to hurt me" or "making a fool of myself" to a more useful stance of what can he do to help himself cope more effectively. Recall that these patients spend their energy thinking about what *might* happen. Thus, the primary type of control we teach the patient is *cognitive.*

As with the problems in Chapter 6 and 7, the key to success with these patients is to help them actively cope with their distress. This changes the patient role from passive recipient to an active partner in treatment and allows a greater measure of control. Existing patient coping skills are recognized and developed further. These patients recognize that they do not cope well with a variety of life's stresses and are asked to try a new, simple technique that might help.

Basic to the clinical skills outlined in this chapter is an understanding of anticipation and its role in fostering anxiety. Then a number of important strategies are offered:

1. Altering expectations

2. Redefining the experience

3. Thought stopping

4. Focusing attention

5. Relaxation training

6. Hypnosis

At the conclusion of this chapter we discuss the passive patient and postoperative problems. Treatment strategies for this type of patient are summarized in Appendix C in the *Treatment Modality Checklist.*

ANTICIPATION

In 1958, Janis investigated the psychological effects of surgery based on the self-report provided by patients, some of whom were routine dental patients. Results indicated that the preoperative fear of normal dental patients was high one day before treatment and even higher than that of general surgical patients an hour before treatment.

There is an excellent example of this phenomenon in the dental literature. A series of careful studies by Shannon and his colleagues makes it clear that marked emotional reactions, as assessed by urinary cortisol, derive mainly from the anticipation of dental procedures. Shannon and Isbell (1963) subjected 258 healthy young men to an injection procedure and, because the men had not been aware they were scheduled for dental work, long-term anticipation was held to a minimum. Five experimental treatments were employed: (1) injection of 2 percent lidocaine HCl; (2) injection of 2 percent lidocaine HCl with epinephrine, 1:100,000; (3) injection of 0.9 percent sodium chloride; (4) needle insertion with no injection; (5) a statement that injection would shortly occur, but no actual injection. In the latter condition, the needle was placed in the mouth but never touched the tissues. This mock injection provided the anticipation condition, a purely psychological procedure.

The results clearly show that all of the experimental conditions produced significant increases in hydrocortisone in the urine. What is particularly interesting is that the mock injection procedure produced as much hormonal increase as any of the other procedures. This demonstrates that expectation produced the full emotional response. Anticipation of harm is present in each of the physical conditions. It may be that this alone accounts for the upset associated with injection and other dental procedures.

Laboratory experiments by Lazarus and his colleagues (1966) provide additional evidence of the important role of anticipation. "Suspense" films showing a sequence of events leading to an industrial accident were compared to a "surprise" film made by excising the footage leading up to the accident. The autonomic arousal, measured by heart rate and skin conductivity, was greater in the suspense group. Moreover, for both films, most of the rise in autonomic functioning occurred *before* the accident; seeing the accident added comparatively little to the reaction that had occurred during anticipation.

Jackson (1978), at the Behavioral Science Laboratory of the University of Florida College of Dentistry, provided evidence of the importance of anticipation. Questionnaires about fearful dental events were completed by over 600 individuals. It was not surprising that high and low fear patients' perception of various dental situations differed. The disproportionate fear in phobic patients seemed to center on anticipating events, i.e., "calling the dentist to make an appointment," "sitting in the dentist's waiting room," and "getting in the dentist's chair."

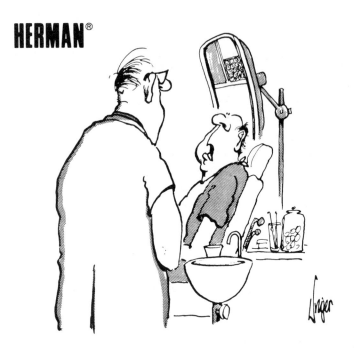

HERMAN®

"Why did your nurse want to know my 'next-of-kin'?"

ORIGINS OF ANTICIPATORY ANXIETY

Reiss (1980) theorizes that anticipatory anxiety occurs in many patients because the patient experiences either *in vivo* or covert associations between the feared stimulus and anxiety. The patient may also be afraid of becoming anxious. That is, if the physiological arousal associated with the label of anxiety is very persuasive, the anticipation of the anxiety could itself become fear eliciting. MacLean (1967) has shown that under such conditions the brain's electrical activity is temporarily altered.

Anticipation has a thought as well as an arousal component. What we tell ourselves in such situations usually increases our arousal. Dysfunctional thoughts or self-statements usually predict catastrophic events and emerge as though they are by reflex—without any prior reflection or

216

reason. At times a vivid sequence of events presents itself, such as having a cardiac arrest and dying in the dental chair. Often just a few words or a brief visual image, e.g., "can't stand it" or visualization of a large needle or other trauma-inducing instrument. Negative events need not only involve trauma. Many catastrophizing patients also fear embarrassment. "What if they think I'm crazy by being so fearful . . . they will laugh at my fear behind my back." These dysfunctional thoughts are hard to turn off. They seem to come and go with a will of their own. Moreover, no matter how irrational, they are always believed and taken seriously by the patient. We have all read the childhood story of the little train that could. These patients are the little *train* that *could not*.

The remainder of this chapter deals with the following concepts: (1) altering expectations by (a) redefining successful experiences, (b) redefining the experience; (2) thought stopping, and (3) focusing attention through (a) calling up existing skills, (b) distraction, (c) relaxation training, and (d) hypnosis. In the last part of the chapter, we will discuss the non-coping patient, and various pharmacologic approaches which may be successful in helping them receive treatment.

ALTERING EXPECTATIONS

The Importance of Redefining Success and Offering Praise

Our observations of fearful persons have led to the realization that small methodical steps are required for these patients to overcome their difficulties. However, characteristic of these individuals is the desire for a "magic bullet" or quick solution. This is why so many initially seek care under general anesthetic when they come to see us. Do not allow patient pressure for an unrealistically quick solution to alter *your* behavior.

Because of the tendency to want a quick solution, these patients need praise at each step of treatment. For example, we treated a patient in the Dental Fears Research Clinic who had severe periodontal disease. The treatment involved repeated root planing and curettage under local anesthetic. We taught the patient a relaxation exercise and he practiced it for a week before his first injection and treatment. The dental hygienist spent several minutes having the patient practice the relaxation procedure and then administered an infiltration injection.

Afterwards the following occurred:

Patient: Whew! I'm glad that's over. I still felt anxious during the injection.

Hygienist: Of course, but you managed very well.

Patient: Yes, but I feel embarrassed to have to sit up. It seems silly.

Hygienist: Overcoming these fears takes time and patience. You did extremely well. I am happy for you. The practicing of the relaxation exercises you did last week really paid off. Shall we proceed?

The scaling was then carried out successfully.

Positive reinforcement and praise can take other forms. Some patients are afraid of the rubber dam. In this case, we will schedule time to practice applying the dam on an anterior tooth to try breathing through the nose and swallowing. Patients are taught to operate the suction and allowed to use it whenever needed. We ask the patient to tell us when he feels he has mastered the skill and provide lots of praise when the skill is acquired. A warm, caring demeanor is appropriate with this patient. Reassurance and encouragement are really useful.

Some patients may not respond to praise the first time. Several visits may be necessary to overcome their doubts of self-efficacy or perceived inability to master the coping. Do not promise complete success, such as completion of a feared procedure, by a certain appointment. With frequent praise and repeated attempts, they will master the skill they need and feel good about themselves. Note: no matter how small the step forward, we all need feedback about our performance in order to improve. Positive "strokes" really work. The anxious patient may continue to discount his or her progress and still desire a quick solution.

On the other hand, some patients are completely preoccupied with their imminent or actual discomfort. Initially, they are unwilling to focus on anything else. It appears that their attention is on discomfort; all reports are negative. For such patients, slowly broaden their attention so that it includes non-negative events. Helping these patients recognize and verbalize neutral and positive perceptions is crucial.

Fordyce (1976) presents techniques for chronic pain patients which have utility for the dental patient. After establishing rapport, Fordyce recommends redirecting attention toward desired perceptions and verbalizations and ignoring maladaptive patient constriction of attention. Modeled on this, we reinforce attention to positive or neutral verbalizations and praise positive patient self-reports of progress. Less and less reinforcement is given for negative comments. For example, debriefings after a session may proceed as follows:

Dentist: How did it go?

Patient: Well . . . it was terrible! You said you wouldn't hurt me, but when you put on the rubber dam you pinched me twice . . . and when you. . . .

Dentist: OK, now, can you recall a moment when you were feeling okay?

Patient: Let me think. . . .

Dentist: At this point in your treatment, please pay as much attention as you can to what is going right, not wrong, with your treatment. Don't let negative thoughts store up; let me know as soon as they happen.

The Importance of Redefining the Experience

Expectations have a dual effect, facilitating the entry of certain stimuli and inhibiting others. When more than one stimulus falls upon receptors at the same time, the one we are prepared for has an advantage and gains entry. Once the response is under way, the other reponses are blocked. This is true not only for pain but also for other sensations.

Patient expectation is capable of influencing whether and how sensations are experienced. Anticipation of what is to follow will itself influence the experience. In a study of experimentally induced pain (Chaves and Barber, 1974), subjects who were led by researchers to expect a reduction in pain compared to their initial trial, but who were not provided with a coping strategy, in fact reported a significant reduction in pain. Clinically, there is evidence that expectation can influence positive treatment outcomes. Expectations are communicated both verbally and nonverbally by clinicians and may be the central reason for the success of a clinical technique.

An example of how expectation affects treatment is audioanalgesia. Gardner and Licklider (1959) and Gardner, Licklider, and Weisz (1960) investigated the effectiveness of white noise and music in suppressing dental pain. They reported that music promotes relaxation and that white noise directly suppresses pain. It was not long before other clinicians were using this technique but with mixed results. As Melzack (1973) described it, some dentists and patients achieved dramatic results. With others, it did not work at all. Many dentists quickly became disillusioned. In a controlled laboratory study, Melzack, Weisz, and Sprague (1963) demonstrated that white noise did not abolish the pain of putting a hand in an ice bucket for five minutes (the cold pressor test). They compared three groups of subjects. Group 1 received strong white noise and music but no suggestion about the purpose of stimulation. Group 2 received strong white noise and music together with a suggestion of its effectiveness for reducing pain. Group 3 received suggestion but only a low-frequency control hum. Each group served as its own control, having received ice bucket pain without any sound before and after the experimental condition. Group 2 (noise, music, and suggestion) produced a substantial increase in how long the subjects could keep their hands in the bucket, but Group 1 (noise and music) and Group 3 (control) did not. Expectations of effectiveness are critical.

Another clinical problem involving expectation is the effectiveness of topical anesthetic. Pollack (1960) hypothesized that the expectation of anesthesia by the patient may be the most important factor in obtaining or failing to obtain a painless injection. Comparing a topical anesthetic to placebo under conditions of suggestion versus no suggestion, he found expectation was important in obtaining a more comfortable injection.

Of the four diagnostic groups of fearful patients we identified in Chapter 4, the anxious individual is most open to suggestion, reassurance, and the authority of the health professional. He responds readily to enthusiasm, smiles, and praise, and concern is accepted and appreciated. As suggested in the model of self-efficacy in Chapter 2, this patient *wants* to be cooperative; what he lacks is a belief that what he can do will be effective, or what he does is "good" enough. He sets unrealistically high standards for himself, which he repeatedly fails to meet. These patients have very high avoidance gradients just before visits and are the most likely to cancel and not respond to appointment confirmation calls. As noted above, in beginning to work with this type of patient, it is useful to start by helping him set both realistic expectations and reasonable definitions of success and copying.

THOUGHT STOPPING

Patients are able to control their worrying. This is important, for when frightening thoughts occur, frightening emotions invariably follow. It is helpful to have the anxious patient keep a record of the negative thoughts arising during the interval before the next dental appointment. Just keeping the record will tend to make some patients better. For example:

Patient: I keep getting these thoughts that the drill will slip and cut me. They make me very upset. I can't sleep . . . they are very upsetting . . . and get worse as the appointment gets closer.

Dentist: I understand. Between now and our next appointment I would like you to keep a log of these thoughts. Write them in this notebook (give the log, an inexpensive small notebook, to the patient). Write the date, time, and context of the thought in as much detail as possible. When you write these thoughts down you begin to gain control over them. You are also aware of how they begin and end. This is the first step in controlling these anticipatory thoughts, which are at the core of your problems.

ADDITIONAL STEPS MAY BE NEEDED. The next few steps of the thought-stopping process may or may not be needed. Let us outline a few techniques. Basic to these steps is the patient imagining the stressful thoughts that were most frequently recorded.

Ask the patient to set an alarm or kitchen timer for three minutes. Instruct her to look away, close her eyes, and ruminate on the stressful thoughts. When she hears the alarm, tell her to shout "stop!" or "enough!" You may also ask the patient to wave her hands in disgust, snap her fingers, or stand up. Following about a 30-second interval, if the stressful thought returns, repeat the shouting procedure.

An alternative procedure involves tape recording the patient loudly yelling "stop!" at intermittent intervals (e.g., three minutes, one minute, two minutes, thirty seconds, one minute, etc.). Proceed the same way as with the alarm or timer. *Have the patient yell with the tape.* You may instruct the patient to rewind to the stop messages as much as needed. The recordings are useful in *strenghtening thought control.*

The next step involves eliminating alarms and tape recorders. Ask the patient to ruminate on the stressful thought and to shout "stop!" When the thought has been eliminated on several occasions with shouts, try to interrupt the thought with "stop" or whatever word is needed, in a normal voice. Subsequent sessions will allow control of the thought with the word verbalized in a whisper. The goal of the process is to use a subvocal command to oneself; that is, to imagine hearing "stop!" shouted within one's mind.

The last step of the procedure involves *thought substitution.* In place of the stressful thought, instruct the patient to either utilize existing positive self-statements or help him make up messages to provide himself. Some messages our patients have successfully used are: "You have lots of skills you can use." "Just remember to keep active and do what you have to do," and "Don't worry; worrying won't help." "What is it I am to do?"

Much of the thought-stopping procedure can be done by patients at home. Patient logs should record all activities. Attempts should be made at least twice a week. Little time is required to explain these procedures and to review patient logs and progress.

Failure at initial attempts should not discourage you or your patient. The most stressful thoughts may be difficult to control. Select a less frightening or intense thought to work on while developing proficiency with the technique.

You should point out that this technique takes time. The thought will return, and you will have to eliminate or interrupt it again and again. Each thought must be stifled as it begins and alternative thoughts substituted. Success rarely occurs without some practice.

One last consideration: if "stop!" or another subvocalization is inadequate, you might recommend the patient keep a rubber band unobtrusively around his wrist. When the stressful thought occurs have the patient snap it or pinch himself. Such behaviors reinforce the subvocalization. For further reading consult Rimm and Masters, *Behavior Therapy: Techniques and Empirical Findings*, New York: Academic Press, 1974.

FOCUSING ATTENTION

Attention

Attention itself may exert considerable influence on what we experience as dental patients. We are all capable of focusing our attention on certain kinds of incoming sensory information, to the exclusion of other inputs. Kanfer and Goldfoot (1966) showed attention influenced pain tolerance in the test described earlier involving keeping a hand in an ice bucket. Subjects distracted by viewing slides or watching a clock were able to keep their hands in the ice the longest. This classic study confirmed the common sense notion that attention-demanding stimuli can function as a distraction and diminish pain perception.

The selective focusing of attention is itself subject to influence by prior experience. Many of us learn to daydream when forced by the nature of the situation to be passive. Students turn off a lecturer, and workers on the assembly line think of after-work activities to get through the day. Such selectivity of attention results in greater comfort and allows us to avoid much of an aversive experience. It has survival value and, as such, is repeated in future situations. A few of us have learned, usually through one discipline or another, e.g., auto-hypnosis, meditation or an oriental martial art, to enter into a deeper trancelike state. In such altered states of consciousness, patients are capable of exercising extreme selectivity of attention. With such control, there is ample evidence that extractions and other usually painful dental treatments are possible even without anesthetic. Nevertheless, we strongly recommend you use local anesthesia in these cases.

Practice at home is necessary. As these strategies are practiced, they become automatic. The patient becomes able to focus his attention and thoughts as he wishes. The practice is to teach the patient to gain some control over his cognitive processes and direct them in two ways. One is to refrain from thinking about what *might* happen, by focusing occasionally on what he or she is *actually* experiencing. At the same time, he or she directs thoughts elsewhere by actively participating in cognitive exercises such as relaxation training, which we will discuss later in this chapter. Researchers (Chaves and Brown, 1978) have found that elimination of catastrophic thoughts is sufficient by itself as a coping skill.

Existing Coping Skills

All of us are able to get through stressful situations in our lives. Of course, some do better than others. Some, for example, feel nervous about speaking in front of others and find it useful to imagine thunderous applause to the talk. As we suggested in Chapter 4, a useful question to ask this patient is, "How do you cope with other stressful situations in your life?" Our goal is to illuminate coping techniques the person already uses which can be applied to dentistry. This technique probably will demand attention and causes the patient to focus on something besides the stressful event.

It has become common for cognitive coping strategies to be taught as part of weight control, smoking cessation, martial arts, natural childbirth, or tension reduction programs. These may be meditation, auto-hypnosis, relaxation, or known by various other names. What they have in common is that they encourage the individual to focus on a comfortable imaginary scene following a guided tape recording, or a word phrase, or *mantra* repeated over and over. They may combine these to cue the person to relax. The deep breathing techniques discussed in Chapter 6 can also be used for this purpose.

We suggest you ask anxious patients if they are familiar with one of these techniques. If so, they may be able to use this technique in the dental setting. In our clinical experience, many dental patients have these skills. However, few will know they can and should also be used at the dentist. Your suggestion will come as a welcome relief.

Case Example

Sometime ago we saw a 40-year-old man with severe periodontal disease. His dentition was intact but at high risk for loss of his teeth. He could not tolerate scaling procedures even when numb. He found that he worried constantly about being hurt, the sensations, and feeling foolish. The dental hygienist found that he practiced a martial arts technique but had not thought to use it at the dentist.

She asked the patient to explain what he did.

Patient: When I begin my exercises, I must concentrate deeply on them. I am still, relaxed, and in deep thought. I can block out noises and often am very aware of my breathing.

Dental Hygienist: This is a very valuable technique. If you can practice this skill here, you will find it will compete successfully with negative thoughts you have been having. We have found it requires a warm-up period before each appointment, here in the operatory. We'll ask you to signal us when you are ready.

Patient: What if it doesn't work?

Dental Hygienist: What you will experience, especially the first few times, is that your concentration will be occasionally disturbed by a dental procedure. We will coach you to regain your concentration and wait until you do so. Each time you do this it will become easier.

Distraction

Researchers have found that electronic games and television and taped relaxation instruction can be successful in controlling high levels of fear in both dental and medical patients. For example, watching TV (Venham, 1977), and playing video Ping-Pong (Corah et al., 1979a) have been employed as distraction techniques during drilling. The experimental work of Corah and associates indicates that a distraction strategy is efficacious in comparison to control strategies. The work assessing the effect of tape-recorded relaxation instructions (Corah et al., 1979a,b and 1981) shows a repetitive set of relaxation instructions played 3 to 4 minutes prior to anesthesia and continued until the procedure was completed, was effective in alleviating anxiety. This strategy relies heavily on distraction: that is, the diversion of attention from the dental procedure to both the tape or to various muscle groups. The key is asking the patient to try to choose an *engaging* activity.

Music is one of the most easily utilized distraction techniques. With portable tape players so inexpensive, many patients have taped music, stories, or comedy they find engaging and can bring. In our clinic, the music system (supplied to us generously by Audio Environments, Inc.) is capable of allowing the patient to select from several different channels, and is adaptable to allow playing patients' cassettes through the system. If at all possible, let the patient control the volume. That way it can be used to drown out noises, such as the drill or high speed vacuum.

There are limitations to the effectiveness of distraction. Especially in early visits with this type of patient, the distractor may not completely eliminate the fatalistic ruminations during injections or drilling. Such patients should be counseled to expect such interruptions as normal. They

226

should be allowed to rest briefly and then instructed to return attention to the distractor. Some patients dislike distraction and for these patients another approach, such as the thought stopping we described earlier, may be more effective.

Convincing a patient that distraction will work is sometimes a problem. One approach is the simple cold pressor test or ice bucket described earlier in this chapter. This test is accomplished by asking the patient to place his hand in an ice bucket for 5 minutes. During the test the patient is given a clock to follow the time but otherwise just asked to deal with the cold pain any way they can. Debriefing afterwards, some will tell you they focused on the pain. Others will have made self-statements such as, "I know I can do it," etc. Still others will say they listened to radio or television and the time passed quickly. Information from these tests will help you and your patient to construct a successful distraction strategy. As an aside, it is interesting to note that a brief application of intense cold has an analgesic effect itself (Melzack et al., 1980).

For some patients, it is difficult not to focus on what they imagine might happen. Learning how to alter one's focus of attention is a slow, incremental process. Thus, the provision of distractors may be useful. As an example, airlines have always tried to create a distracting environment. Attractive and attentive personnel, alcohol, hot meals, multichannel stereo music, movies, and magazines available for reading are all part of a successful technique which prevents travelers, many of whom are anxious about flying, from thinking about being encased in a fragile aluminum and plastic tube, 35,000 feet above the ground. Some of the distraction techniques utilized successfully in the dental office are built right into the environment. Decorating offices with nontraditional decor and using space to eliminate sights, sounds, and smells traditionally associated with dentists' offices is a widely used and helpful strategy. Recently, there have been articles about the calming effects of observing tropical fish and windows. In fact, dentists have traditionally used the technique of diverting attention to facilitate child management. Talking to a child about his favorite animal while the child is being examined is an example of this technique. Such techniques can be equally successful with the adult patient.

Relaxation Training

In the previous section, we mentioned that relaxation tapes may prove to be effective in control of anxiety and distress, as they distract the patient from his catastrophic cognitions. Relaxation instructions are different from relaxation training, which takes considerable practice. Clum et al. (1982) presented evidence that the results are different. Relaxation training is more effective in reducing pain-related distress and the verbal report of pain than are simple instructions to "try and relax" without training.

Relaxation training may take many forms. The procedure that has received the most scrutiny is called "progressive relaxation" and was developed by Edmond Jacobson, a Chicago physician, in 1929. The technique is based on the premise that the body responds to anxiety-provoking thoughts and events with muscle tension. This physical tension, in turn, increases the subjective experience of anxiety. Muscle relaxation reduces physiological tension and is incompatible with anxiety. The habit of responding with relaxation blocks anxiety; it is impossible to be physically relaxed and psychologically upset at the same time. Excellent results have been found with this technique in the treatment of a large number of anxiety-implicated problems including insomnia, fatigue, muscle spasm, neck and back pain, stuttering, high blood pressure, and a variety of phobias.

The procedures are simple but require practice. One or two 15-minute sessions a day for one to two weeks are recommended. After a demonstration and supervised practice, patients can practice at home. Ask them to practice at the same time and place and to record their practice sessions in a log. Notations of how they feel before and after each session are useful to you and them in assessing progress.

The following set of instructions has been utilized with our fearful patients. The basic procedure involves tensing specific muscle groups for five to seven seconds immediately followed by 20 seconds of relaxation. The procedure may be demonstrated and practiced in a dental chair. Four major muscle groups are tensed and relaxed one at a time. They are:

1. Hands, forearm, and biceps
2. Feet, calves, thighs, buttocks

3. Chest, stomach, and lower back

4. Head, face, throat, and shoulders

We recommend the clinician initially demonstrate the procedure to the patient with his or her eyes open. An initial 10- to 20-minute session will bring some relaxation. We go through the procedure twice, primarily to demonstrate that practice is valuble in enhancing relaxation. With home practice, it will be possible for the patient to relax in the dental chair in just a few minutes. Making an audio tape of the second time through the procedure and providing it to the patient to play at home is a useful strategy. It is helpful to talk slowly and softly to the patient and to provide suggestion during the relaxation phases.

You may desire to use the following expresssions:

Relax and smooth out the muscles . . .

Let the tension melt away . . .

Loose . . . limp . . . calm . . .

Feel rested . . . calm . . . tension gone . . .

The instructions and procedure we use are as follows:

> Find a comfortable position . . . and relax. Now clench your fists, tighten . . . tighten. Study the tension . . . Notice the tension in your fist and forearm. Now relax. Feel the looseness. Notice the contrast with the tension. Now bend your elbows and tense your biceps . . . as hard as you can. Feel the tautness. . . . Okay, relax, straighten out your arms. Let them hang there loose and limp. Loose and limp, let the relaxation come to you. Feel the difference.
>
> Now let us go to your feet. Curl your toes. Do you feel your calves tense? Good. But don't tense so much that your muscles will cramp. Now relax. Let the tension melt away. Muscles feel loose and limp? Now, bend your toes toward your

face. Feel the tension in your shins. Relax again . . . loose, rested.

Feel the heaviness in your lower body. Relax your knees, thighs and buttocks. Loose . . . limp . . . relaxed. Tension will leave, let it go and melt away. Now let it spread to stomach, lower back and chest. Let go more and more. Deeper, deeper. . . .

Now we will turn our attention to your neck and shoulders. Lots of tension there. Hunch them up and tighten them . . . more. . . . Okay . . . relax. How good it feels. Warm, comfortable, loose and limp. Relaxed. Allow your brow to become smooth again. Notice any strain in your forehead or scalp? Now close your eyes . . . hard! Tighten. Feel the tension. Relax your eyes. You may feel most comfortable with them closed. You are becoming more and more relaxed.

Now clench your jaw, biting hard, lips slightly parted, as if you were angry. Relax. Feel the difference? Notice that your jaw is slightly open. This is a natural, relaxed position. The more relaxed your face and mouth are the easier dentistry will be for you. Good . . . you are doing fine.

Let *all* of your body relax. Enjoy the calm peaceful feeling. Your body is heavy and loose. Relaxed. . . .

At this point we often utilize a rhythmic breathing exercise. Ask the patient to breathe in and completely fill his or her lungs. Have him hold it. Point out the tension. Have him exhale slowly and suggest looseness in the chest. "Hear the slow hiss and continue relaxing. Let your breathing become slow, free, and gentle. Notice even more tension leaving you."

Remember practice is important. Being able to relax quickly is a skill. Demonstrate the skill, have the patient practice at home, and call on the skill. When the patient comes in for the next appointment, seat him in the chair a few minutes early to relax and practice his relaxation and breathing exercise.

The following passages are excerpts from a log one of our patients kept of her practice. You may want to have your patients keep a log like this.

12/1 Start 5:00 P.M.
I was overtired and it was hard to get to sleep, so I did relaxation breathing, listening to very soft music. My body became very relaxed, and like you said, the breathing takes over. I didn't even realize I was breathing. Soon the breathing became almost trancelike. It is an unusual feeling, it seems like someone else is controlling my breathing. As I went along further it seemed like my breathing slowed down considerably. I stopped at about 5:13 and slept only about 4 and a half hours, but it felt like a whole night.

12/2 4:30 A.M.
Our computer system at work went down and we lost all the work that was keyed in since 11:00 P.M., and I was working with our Engineer over the phone to get the system up. This was very upsetting because I knew that I would have to work Saturday to make up the work and I really had my heart set on going to Leavenworth. Put it this way, I was upset and under a lot of stress. During my lunch at 4:30 I laid down and did the muscle exercises which helped a lot and then I did the breathing. When my lunch was through I went back to work feeling relaxed and ready to tackle the work. The rest of the morning went fine. When I left work and went outside and saw snow it made my day. I don't need to go to the mountains for snow. Begin time 4:30; end 5:00.

12/4 2:00 P.M.
Muscle tensing and relaxing really help but I have a way where I focus completely on various parts of my body and cause them to relax. I usually start from my feet and up and out to my hands. I did this and then the breathing. The breathing gives me a feeling of warmth and heaviness like nitrous oxide does.

Almost I am sinking further and further. It is very relaxing. At times I want to go to sleep after. Other times I have so much energy. Start 2:00; end 2:30

12/5 4:00 A.M.
I was having extremely bad menstrual cramps so I laid down. I decided to do the relaxation and breathing. It helped, aspirin usually doesn't even work. End 4:30

During the day off and on I will just breathe deeply. It is becoming so natural. I wish it would help the tendonitis that is getting worse.

12/8
I have been doing the exercises twice daily but the writing is not so regular. Start 3:00 p.m. One of the easiest and most relaxing times is before I go to sleep. Today wasn't very successful. When I was really in a relaxed state, the paper slammed against the door, a very rude awakening. Started over again but couldn't get into it. End 3:15 p.m.

12/9
A day off from work for me. Shopped all day so I was ready for some relaxation. Start 8:30. I am repeating myself but the exercises are so relaxing. My body gets so warm and heavy like I am floating. Ending time I don't know, I fell asleep.

We recommend Bernstein and Borkovec's, little book, *Progressive Relaxation Training: A Manual for the Helping Professional* (Champaign, Illinois, Research Press, 1973) for those who would like more information and a slightly different approach.

Hypnosis

In the last three decades, there has been growing clinical application of hypnosis. Dentists, physicians, and psychologists have utilized a wide variety of hypnotic techniques. Case histories and descriptions of successful pain control using hypnosis are common not only in dentistry, but in obstetrics, internal medicine, cardiology, dermatology, and psychiatry. There are well-established journals, for example the *International Journal of Clinical and Experimental Hypnosis* and the *American Journal of Clinical Hypnosis*, numerous medical texts, and continuing dental and medical education courses teaching hypnotic technque.

But what is hypnosis? How does it work? There are a number of theories. Chaves and Barber (1974) have argued, and we agree, that the success of hypnosis is primarily based upon the patient's acceptance of suggestion. It is not based on powers certain individuals have to influence others.

With hypnotic induction, suggestions are made that certain physiological effects (such as bodily relaxation) will occur. Rapport and trust are established. Subjects are silent and often are asked to close their eyes. Each of these variables contributes to produce a person who is more apt to accept the suggestion of comfort. According to Barber (1965), much of what is done under hypnosis could also be done with the patient awake. According to the results of experiments on this subject by Lazarus (1971), the "effectiveness of the therapy is closely linked with ... expectations."

There are other theories of why hypnosis works (Hilgard, 1973). However, such theories are of relatively little use to the dental clinician. What is most important is that the dental treatment done under hypnosis for the patient with generalized anxiety could probably not be done as easily without it or some similar technique. The anxiety-related behaviors, and failure to exert cognitive control, would result in failed appointments and treatment complications. The hypnotic approach, just as local anesthesia, is a tool to be used in the care of certain patients.

Hypnosis has a stage-show connotation about it; and as such, many clinicians are reluctant to learn these techniques. Although it is beyond the scope of this text to teach hypnotic technique, the following example should help the reader understand its potent effect and stimulate further interest in learning the clinical skills. This technique is appropriate with the particular kind of patient discussed in this chapter because they are often trusting and willing to accept the authority of a professional.

Case Example

This 35-year-old woman was seen in the Dental Fears Research Clinic with extensive inflammation in the gingiva surrounding an anterior crown. The situation was exacerbated by traumatic occlusion. Otherwise, the patient's condition was normal. Assessment revealed anxiety about treatment as well as other psychological concerns outside dentistry.

The treatment began at the initial consultation visit. The patient was asked if she could daydream. She said she could. She was placed in a comfortable position and asked to close her eyes and daydream. This exercise was to teach her skills she could use in the dental chair: no dental treatment was to be accomplished this visit.

After beginning to daydream, she was taught to signal with a finger raised thus avoiding distracting conversation. Then she was asked to take a series of long, full breaths, and as she exhaled, immerse herself more and more deeply in her reverie. After about five breaths, she was asked in a low, calm voice to focus on the various senses during her daydream. For example, if she was walking in the woods, to try to imagine the color of the sky, the smell of the trees, the feeling of the wind, etc. At each step, she would signal that she was able. At the same time, suggestion was given that this is a good feeling that can be used in any situation that is stressful. After 15 minutes of practice, alertness is regained by reversing the process. Breathing concentrates on inhalation and in a louder, faster voice she was asked by the clinician to be alert. Praise was given for completing this exercise, and the patient reported feeling quite good. Homework exercises involving practice were provided.

On the next visit, the hypnotic state was reached within 5 minutes. This time numbness is added to the repertory of feelings imagined. "Try to imagine your foot going to sleep. It may feel heavy and numb yet not uncomfortable . . . perhaps you can feel this same sensation in your hand or lip. . . ."

Then topical and infiltration anesthesia were easily and effectively administered. Post-hypnotic suggestion left the patient alert and with a skill to deal well with a previously feared experience.

PATIENTS WHO INSIST ON A PASSIVE ROLE

We have enountered some anxious patients for whom these approaches do not work as well as required. These stem less from misdiagnosis than from our inability to help this patient to take an active role in his or her own care. That is, some patients perceive that their comfort and experience are *completely* the responsibility of dental personnel. They do not believe they have a role in coping with the experience. They will not do their homework or practice the skills while at the dentist, and refuse to believe they can do anything to help themselves. The clinical problem is non-coping. A typical conversation with this type of patient might sound like this:

Dentist: You dealt with the fillings today very well.

Patient: I don't think so. It was just like all the other times.

Dentist: What do you mean?

Patient: The fillings were just unbearable. I don't think I can go through with it again.

These patients are frustrating to work with because they have such negative attitudes. Persistence and patience are essential for treating this patient; however, pharmacologic approaches may be useful adjuncts. The two we regularly employ in the Dental Fears Research Clinic are nitrous oxide and oxygen and oral premedication. These patients may also be candidates for IV sedation. When these drugs are used in conjunction with the cognitive strategies discussed earlier, such patients can be successfully treated. A more detailed discussion of these medications, their advantages and limitations, is in Chapter 3.

COMPLIANCE WITH POST-OPERATIVE INSTRUCTIONS

In our experience we have found some of our general anxiety patients are paralyzed by their thoughts to the extent they do not follow post-operative instructions. One patient was so exhausted from the emotion of her dental visit she failed to take her antibiotics four times per day. She persisted in only taking three tablets per day even though it was suggested she could alter the drug schedule to suit her routine.

Another patient called the evening after a procedure during the day to say he was in pain. Inquiry found he had failed to pick up the prescription for pain medicine. In such patients, it's very difficult to interpret these responses. For such a patient, the use of anti-inflammatory drugs and long acting anesthetics maybe helpful (Dionne et al., 1984).

For patients in this diagnostic category we recommend written post-operative instructions.

CONCLUSION

This chapter is about treatment of the anxious dental patient with generalized anxiety. This is the patient who anticipates problems and often cannot find a way to cope. We offer two general approaches. First, we alter expectations by redefining success and the nature of the dental experience. Second, we focus attention through the use of existing coping skills, distraction, relaxation training, hypnosis, and other skills.

QUESTIONS AND EXERCISES

1. To illustrate the role of anticipation, think back to the last time you experienced some significant anxiety, such as, the last important examination that you took. What bodily responses can you remember? What

did you think of before the actual experience? As it turned out, did you need to worry ahead of time? Were you able to talk yourself out of the feelings? If so, what did you tell yourself? If not, what could you have done differently?

2. Describe how you would recommend a friend overcome negative, anticipatory, and catastrophizing thoughts.

3. List as many distractors as you can think of that might conceivably be adapted to use in the dental operatory. Start with as many as you can; brainstorm, listing everything that comes to mind.

4. Recall some of the patients or other people you have known. What are some of their characteristics, qualities, abilities that they had used to overcome fearful situations?

NINE

Treatment of the Patient Who Is Afraid of Catastrophe

GENERAL CONSIDERATIONS

These patients focus their attention on bodily sensations. Just as general anxiety patients (see Chapter 8) cannot manage to control their fearful thoughts, these patients are preoccupied with some possible malfunction of their body. Knowledge of the patient's locus of attention is the key to successful diagnosis and treatment.

The key fear of these patients is the fear response itself—the panic of being out of control. Some are simply afraid they will have an emotional anxiety attack. Most are anxious that they will experience a traumatic physical reaction. These patients are afraid of a catastrophe such as a stroke, heart attack, or choking to death. They may be convinced they are allergic to lidocaine or epinephrine, or that dentist error will result in severe injury. Ironically, though stricken with panic, many do not think of themselves as being fearful. Fear may be denied or seen as secondary. They are often capable of discussing problems with their body in a very logical and thoughtful manner. The problem usually centers on fear of a specific procedure. For example, fear of choking to death with a rubber dam in place falls in this category. These patients may have had considerable dental treatment, some quite recently. Treatment strategies are outlined in the *Treatment Modality Checklist* found in Appendix C.

ORIGIN OF THE FEAR

There are two complementary conceptualizations that help explain how an individual experiencing dental fear becomes emotionally upset. They are especially useful in understanding patients who are afraid of catastrophe. The first theory is outlined as follows:

Environmental stimulus $\rightarrow$ physiological arousal $\rightarrow$ upset, e.g., fear.

Case Example

An example of a patient who typifies this categorization is Mrs. Susan. In childhood, she became afraid of numbness. She reported being fearful that the numbness from local anesthetic would spread throughout her body and she would not "wake up." The stimulus of the anesthetic numbness results in arousal. Negative thoughts about the significance of those sensations lead to upset and panic. Simply put, the theory behind this formulization claims: *The emotions we experience depend on the label we place on the arousal felt inside our bodies.*

The second conceptualization looks at the upset of patients as follows:

Environmental stimulus → negative thoughts → physiological arousal → upset, e.g., fear.

In theory two, an environmental stimulus, e.g., rubber dam, leads to negative thoughts ("I won't be able to breathe"), followed by physiological arousal (which includes apparent respiratory difficulty), and an extreme panic response.

In 1962, Schachter and Singer conducted a classic experiment that has greatly influenced how psychologists view emotions. They administered epinephrine by injection to a subject who was told that it was Suproxin, a new vitamin compound. The subject was then placed in a waiting room for 15 to 20 minutes. A stooge, supposedly just Suproxin injected, was brought in to pass the waiting time with the subject. A short while after the injection, the subject experienced typical nervous system arousal: hand tremors, heart pounding, and rapid breathing. As the drug took effect, the stooge began behaving in one of two ways. He either became progressively more angry or he became increasingly euphoric. During this period the subject was watched through a two-way mirror and his behavior was observed and systematically recorded. It was found that subjects who had waited with the angry stooge became angry, and those who waited with the euphoric stooge became euphoric. Subjects with a saline placebo had no emotional reaction, no matter how the stooge functioned. Subjects who were warned in advance that Suproxin sometimes will have side effects of trembling and heart pounding had no emotional reaction, regardless of the stooge's behavior.

Schachter made the following conclusions from his experiment:

1. Emotion is not merely a chemical reaction that automatically creates feelings. Physiological arousal, by itself, cannot produce specific emotions.

2. A state of physiological arousal for which the subject has no immediate explanation makes him want to understand it. He will actively search his environment for an appropriate explanation or "label" for the arousal. Choice of labels will determine the emotional response.

A specific emotion is, at least in part, created by evaluation of internal and external events. Subjects in the study attributed their arousal to either anger or euphoria depending on what appeared to be appropriate, based on the emotional reaction of the stooge.

Schacter's study has important implications for treating emotional upset. It suggests that patients become anxious, for example, by saying certain things to themselves. They attribute their physiological arousal to the emotion of fear and consequently interpret something in their environment as implying danger. This interpretation can be made by seeing something that seems threatening or noticing that someone else is afraid and believing that there must be good reason for alarm. *Emotion depends on thought.* Thought precedes emotion. If the attributions and interpretations can be changed, so can the distressing emotion. Health professionals influence these thoughts. For example, there are clinical reports of fearful patients who, when told that arousal (e.g., increased heart beat) was caused by the epinephrine in the anesthetic and not their fear, became much less fearful. On the other hand, it is our impression that clinicians often attribute fear related responses to drug reactions.

Panic Disorders and Attribution

Recent research by David Sheehan (1980, 1982) and others indicate that frightening though minor medical conditions such as: heart pounding, tachycardia, light-headedness, nausea, rubbery legs, choking sensations, etc., may be caused by an underlying biochemical abnormality or cardio-vascular pathology (mitral valve prolapse) and are responsible for some cases of panic disorders. This has been categorized as endogenous anxiety. When organic causes are not found upon consultation with physicians, the problem may be attributed to a lack of sanity which results in addi-tional symptoms; or it may be attributed, or conditioned to events and sit-uations (such as dentistry) associated with these panic attacks. To avoid these attacks, patients may begin to avoid many situations. In our clinical experience, we have found patients can be taught to "decondition" them-selves, and learn to identify initial symptoms that allow them to short cir-cuit the panic reaction in its early phases.

Cognitive theorists Beck (1979) and Ellis (1975) are the leading pro-ponents of theory two. They argue that emotional reactions are a result of the way we structure reality. If patients are anxious, they suggest it is be-cause they are interpreting events as dangerous. If a patient is depressed, it is because he sees himself as defective or the victim of loss. Anger is pro-duced by perceptions that one is suffering abuse and is a victim of injus-tice. *Each painful emotion is created by a particular negative thought.*

Chronic upset is the by-product of a systematic bias in viewing the world. To the "depressive," for example, every event is an opportunity to see himself in some way diminished. Then he gets the "sinking feeling" in his stomach, which he labels depression. The anxious person tends to view even innocuous events as threatening. Many of our patients even fear the rubber prophy cup. These threats set off the "fight or flight" alarm responses, which he labels anxiety.

These two theories of emotion cited indicate the importance of pa-tient thought in the fear response. The theories are complementary and both help to explain the behavior of our patients in this diagnostic cate-gory. Moreover, these theories have importance in treatment as well. The patient has responsibility too; he is not just a victim of previous condi-tioning. The way he labels or evaluates the situation in the future determines his emotional reactions. The dentist, in treating the fear, has responsibility for influencing the labeling done by the patient.

ALTERING ATTRIBUTION

The first step in treating these patients involves altering their perception of the problem. To explain this, let us look at a problem involving an adverse reaction to local anesthetic. It is not uncommon for a patient or the dentist to attribute a reaction to a drug. Patients tell us that they have had adverse reactions to the epinephrine in the anesthetic. Dentists are often convinced and convince these patients that the source of the problem is drug related.

An experiment by Valins (1966) provides more clues about how these responses evolve. In his experiment, subjects were shown slides of Playboy nudes while supposedly listening to their heart rates. In fact, they were listening to a recording of a heartbeat, the rate of which could be manipulated to speed up or slow down. For half of the slides, subjects heard their "heart rate" increase. These slides were later rated by these subjects as more attractive than slides for which the heart rate did not change. Valins explained this finding by suggesting that subjects convinced themselves that a slide was attractive by actively searching for attributes that might have caused such a dramatic heart rate increase.

The same researcher, with a colleague, found in a 1967 study that subjects were more apt to approach a live snake if led to believe that their heart rates had not increased while watching the snake. What Valins showed was that *emotional response can depend on what you think your internal state is* regardless of what is actually going on inside your body. Once again thought is the prerequisite for emotion. Occasionally, we monitor the heart rate of fearful patients in the dental chair. Telling the patient in reassuring tones that his heart rate is "steady" and that he is doing very well seems to result in lowered heart rate.

In the simplest clinical case, it is possible to explain to the patient the real cause of his heart palpitations and give him informational control over the events at the dentist. Imagine this interaction:

Dentist: The anesthetic drug we are using has some normal side effects you need to understand.

Patient: OK.

Dentist: Mainly you may feel your pulse quicken or even some chest pounding for a few moments.

Patient: Is this dangerous?

Dentist: No, it is normal and will pass very soon.

With a patient who is afraid of a drug reaction, you may want a different attribution strategy where the reaction is attributed to normal physiological responses:

Dentist: Have you noticed when you think about receiving an injection that you begin to sweat?

Patient: Yes.

Dentist: This is a normal physiological response to feeling anxious.

Patient: I am worried that I am having a reaction to the drug.

Dentist: These drugs we use have almost no side-effects. What you feel should be interpreted as related to anxiety, not drugs.

Though such simple explanations should be attempted, they may not be sufficient to alter patient fear-related responses, especially for those who do not recognize that they are fearful. For these patients we provide the "broken toaster message" to establish that we understand their problem. It goes something like this:

> I know you must feel like a person who has placed a piece of bread in a toaster and almost was electrocuted. Sparks flying everywhere. You take the toaster to an expert . . . the small appliance repairman . . . and he checks it out with his instruments and tells you that everything is really okay. What do you do?

Do you dare use the toaster again? Just because he did not find anything wrong does not mean the situation is not dangerous.

Most patients understand the metaphor and the empathy that you generate at this point is gratefully appreciated. It will allow you to proceed: the next step involves a careful examination of the "toaster" by both of you.

Case Example

Another case involved Mr. Green who feared death in the dental chair. He searched out the emergency oxygen in the operatory and repeatedly asked about emergency precautions. He presented with severe periodontal disease and some broken restorations. Our primary strategy involved structuring his visits so short procedures could be accomplished successfully and providing rest breaks to allow the patient control over the pace of treatment. The patient often felt the need to sit up after an injection. When more than one injection was required, rest breaks were programmed in between the injections. These rest breaks allowed Mr. Green to "calm down" and reduce his physiological arousal level before proceeding further—thus reducing his fears, "that things will begin to run out of control."

It is critical to note that we do not deny that patients experience their particular physical reaction. Instead, we provide praise for surviving even though they felt physical upset. These patients will frequently deny that their coping techniques are working and repeatedly need to be helped to learn to control the reaction that they fear will snowball into panic. We tell the patient that his task is to learn to recognize the initial symptoms indicating that he is about to have a "reaction" and use his coping skill to break the chain of events early on. "Once you are in the middle, it is difficult to control or stop it."

In more difficult cases, we try to demonstrate that we can recreate the

247

symptoms in the dental environment, tachycardia, or dyspnea, without any treatment. This helps to concretely demonstrate to the patient that there is a direct connection between his thoughts and physiological reactions. For many this is an important revelation, and acts as a key to help them learn to control something they once thought was beyond their conscious control. We place the patient in the dental chair and attach a biofeedback monitor, usually a pulse rate monitor that is worn on the earlobe. After some relaxation and breathing instruction, we attempt to have the patient imagine the fearful situation. Patient awareness that the problem is not strictly physical in nature usually occurs at this point. We explain that their re-creation of the feared response is a function of "psychophysiological conditioning," which we will attempt to alter together.

Case Example

The following case history involving a drug reaction illustrates the point: Mrs. Smith, a healthy 40-year-old mother and a health professional herself, came to us seeking assistance with her suspected adverse reactions to local anesthetic. She reported that reactions began five years before while being treated at her current dentist's office. The reactions were reported to begin 20 minutes after injection and were characterized by "tachycardia and a drop in blood pressure." The most recent episode resulted in the emergency involvement of a physician, who told her she had reacted to the epinephrine in the anesthetic. This occurred after she was treated symptomatically for syncope. The patient subsequently had tests for allergy to the anesthetic and preservative: results were negative.

On the surface the patient did not appear fearful. On the other hand, she reported her life is hectic. Her husband noted that she appeared "shaky" a few days prior to dental visits. At the initial therapeutic session, we discussed attribution and her difficulty in accepting that she is not in danger from the anesthetic. She sat vertically in the dental chair and clipped on the lead from a pulsemeter with a digital readout (Sears 629151). After a resting heart rate in the mid-70s was established, she was asked to visualize successively making a dental appointment, approaching the dental office, and being seated in the dental chair. Her heart rate rose from the mid-70s to the mid-80s when visualizing making an appointment, and went up and stayed in the mid-90s when approaching and being seated in the dentist's office. At that point she was asked to "relax." Her response was that her heart rate rose to over 130 bpm and she reported hot flashes and feeling "flushed and panicky." Subsequent discussion revealed a family history of heart disease and that certain thoughts and situations triggered a panic-like response mimicking a heart attack. With these insights, Mrs. Smith began to accept that her mind influenced her physiology. A treatment giving her control over her physiological reaction, namely biofeedback, could now be instituted.

After the patient recognizes the role of thought in his or her physiological response to dental treatment, one of two treatment modalities is presented in our clinic. We either utilize systematic desensitization or biofeedback. These techniques will work with somatic reaction of many types.

SYSTEMATIC DESENSITIZATION

Wolpe's (1958) systematic desensitization was one of the most encouraging developments in psychology in the last generation. In essence, this technique involves substituting a relaxation response for an anxiety response. The presentation of feared stimuli are presented gradually, the least feared stimuli is presented first.

Sample Dental Fear Hierarchy

Imagine:

Making an appointment
Going to the dental office

Sitting in the waiting room

Entering the operatory

Sitting in the chair

Seeing the dentist

Hearing the noises . . .

Receiving an injection

Drilling

This method of treatment has a long and successful history. Mary Cover Jones first reported using the procedure to treat a child who was very afraid of rabbits. She gradually moved the feared object closer and closer to the child while the child was preoccupied eating a favorite food. The strategy of substituting a non-fearful for a fearful response was capitalized upon by Joseph Wolpe who used a simplified version of Jacobson's progressive relaxation training as the non-fearful response. Wolpe's technique included the generation of a hierarchy of fear-producing situations for each patient, specific to the particular fear. The patient is taught to relax and then visualize a scene from the low fear end of the hierarchy. While maintaining the relaxed state, the patient systematically progresses through all items in the hierarchy. After this, patients are able to calmly face the previously frightening situations. Wolpe's method, presented in *Psychotherapy by Reciprocal Inhibition* (1958), has met with considerable success. It has been applied to a wide range of fears. Variations in the technique have been reported. There is evidence, for example, that exposure to real stimuli (*in vivo* desensitization) has succeeded after failure with imaginal desensitization. In our experience, for fearful dental patients, the *in vivo* treatment appears to be as successful as it is with other monosymptomatic phobias (Yates, 1970).

The treatment of dental fear using systematic desensitization can be traced to the work of Gale and Ayer in 1969. Since then many case histories utilizing a variety of desensitization techniques have been reported in the literature (e.g., Klepac, 1975).

Case Examples

An example of a problem solved using *in vivo* desensitization was panic in response to injections: needle phobia. The now adult patient had many traumatic childhood experiences and bringing the syringe to the mouth brought on violent head movement, and grasping the syringe. In treatment the patient was first exposed to the needle with the cover on and asked to practice a deep sighing breath when it was presented near the mouth. This response was practiced first near the mouth, then inside the mouth and repeated over several visits. At first, the panic occurred. Later the sigh became easier and replaced the panic. Then the process was repeated with the needle cover removed. Then, with the patient's permission an injection was given. The sigh replaced the panic, and no uncontrollable movements occurred.

A second example involves a patient whose panic involved gagging and fear of choking. The patient was referred by her dentist because she was unable to tolerate treatment of an upper second molar with dental caries. Attempts to obtain a periapical radiograph had failed repeatedly. The dentist sent along only a panoramic film.

Classical systematic desensitization technique was used to allow the patient to vividly recreate the sensation of gagging outside the dental chair. Thus, it was decided to first recreate the sensation and teach the patient an alternative to panic. In this case, relaxation (and deep breathing) was the preferred response since gagging is caused by muscle tension. As the patient was able to imagine and relax, we moved to the clinic in a series of small graduated steps.

For radiographs, first we worked in the front of the mouth. At each step we practiced the relaxation response. Then over the space of two short appointments we were able to obtain the film. The patient was given homework, i.e., asked to practice relaxation response daily between sessions.

The same approach was used with the rubber dam. Repeated practice at each location, anterior to posterior, produced awareness and mastery. Constant praise, and lots of feedback (e.g., length of time the rubber dam was on) was very helpful. Again, the speed of exposure depends on

251

the progress the patient is making. There is no way to know in advance whether the treatment will take one or two or even six or seven sessions.

Biofeedback

Within Wolpe's technique is the essence of a far-reaching idea—the view that man may acquire voluntary control over a variety of physiological functions, and, in doing so, alter his psychological state. The idea itself is not original. It can easily be traced to eastern disciplines such as Yoga and Zen, and recent therapies such as progressive relaxation and autogenic training.

At the present time, three interesting developments may prove to extend the range and power of this approach: the rapid growth and proliferation of inexpensive electronic instrumentation; research involving events previously found difficult to measure; and the attempt to identify psychophysiological pathways or feedback loops. The electronic measurement of a physiological event and the conversion of the electronic signal to visual, auditory, or some other form of comprehensible feedback allows continuous awareness of a physiological state. This is the essence of biofeedback. Awareness of physiological events not previously attended to by the patient allows the acquisition of voluntary control over physiological functions, many of which were previously considered totally involuntary. Recognition of the learned nature of visceral and glandular function has been especially important. The mechanism by which the CNS influences bodily functions, called "somatization" and "conversion" in previous decades is being uncovered (Miller, 1969).

As a result of the above developments, there have been advances in research and treatment primarily in stress-related disorders. Numerous articles using biofeedback in the treatment of tension and migraine headache, muscle pains, irritable bowel syndrome, insomnia, essential hypertension, Raynauld's disease, etc., are now in the current medical literature. Even the dental literature has a number of citations of the utility of this approach in treatment of myofacial pain-dysfunction syndrome, clenching and bruxism (Solberg and Rugh, 1972; Carlsson et al, 1975; Karduchi and Clarke, 1977; Butler et al., 1976). *Biofeedback and Dentistry: Research and Clinical Applications,* edited by Rugh and others, presents a number of informative papers on the topic.

Biofeedback has been used to treat dental fear. Hirschman and his colleagues (1979, 1980, 1982) have provided evidence that a variety of biofeedback procedures can be useful in the management of dental fear. Using electromyographic (EMG) feedback, Hirschman (1980), in a single brief session, trained dental patients to decrease muscle activity in the forearm. Highly anxious patients who received biofeedback were less anxious during treatment and reported restorative dental treatment as less stressful than anticipated. Highly anxious control group patients, on the other hand, showed increases in anxiety and reported procedures as more stressful than anticipated. Similarly, Hirschman and his colleagues (1979) studied the effects of a simple procedure called "paced respiration." When highly anxious patients use a light signal to pace their respiration at a slower-than-normal rate, they rate dental treatment as less unpleasant than control patients who breathe at a normal or faster-than-normal rate. Promising results were also reported in this paper for heart rate feedback. In fact, Oliver and Hirschman (1982) reported that high dentally anxious subjects exposed to heart rate biofeedback reported less unpleasantness and showed lower heart rates in response to viewing videotapes of stressful dental procedures than did subjects provided with relaxation instructions (see Chapter 8) or those in a control situation.

Clearly, biofeedback offers promise. The procedure is especially useful for those patients who do not recognize their own anxiety, or who believe their bodies may "go out of control" during dental treatment. The procedures are efficient and can be utilized by a dental auxiliary. Moreover, minimal equipment is needed and reliable instruments are widely available at a reasonable cost. A good overview for the student or clinician interested in biofeedback is *Biofeedback: Principles and Practice for Clinicians,* edited by J.V. Basmajian. An additional source may be your local Biofeedback Society or the Biofeedback Society of America (4301 Owens Street, Wheat Ridge, Colorado 80033).

Case Example

The following example illustrates how biofeedback may be used to assist in treatment of patients who fear catastrophe—in this case, allergic reaction to lidocaine.

Mrs. Smith discussed earlier in this chapter accepted that her response was not induced by the anesthetic but was a result of her fearful response to dental treatment. We utilized the pulsemeter, which functioned very well as an assessment tool, and as the major vehicle of her treatment. The goal was to identify and practice a response that would take the place of her anxiety. After instructions and 15 minutes of practice she took the device home and practiced lowering her heart rate for at least 15 minutes every day.

She recorded the time she spent with the device, her heart rate, and subjective responses in a daily log. After identifying a way to maintain her heart rate at the lowest possible point (she began with a resting heart rate in the 80s and ended 10 weeks later with a resting heart rate ten beats per minute lower), she imagined stressful dental and non-dental scenes while she practiced her "calming" response, which relied heavily on control of her respiration. At week eight, the patient was given, in the context of providing dental treatment, half a carpule of anesthetic, with epinephrine. The patient, pulsemeter attached, responded to the placement of the topical anesthetic gel with a 50 beat per minute increase in her heart rate—to over 140 bpm. The patient noted that this was just like her previous episode in her dentist's office. Two subsequent appointments for restorative dentistry were uneventful, with the exception of one period of upset with increased heart rate just about 20 minutes after the injection. The patient pointed out to us that she was still somewhat conditioned to respond anxiously. At this point she had an insight as to why her reaction occurred 20 minutes after the injection. This was about the time her dentist returned to the operatory to begin treatment. Mystery solved!

Relapse

It is important that the alternative responses to panic situations be overlearned or repeatedly practiced. This means the dentist or therapist needs to review basic skills, usually in the waiting room or in the chair prior to treatment. Devote at least a few minutes to practice at each session.

At recall appointments after 3–6 months, the appropriate responses may need considerable rehearsal and practice. Although anxiety will not return to its earlier level, it will be higher on recall than when the last course of treatment finished. At such appointments we take at least fifteen minutes to reestablish our contact with patients, listen to their description of their current anxiety level, and practice or rehearse an appropriate response. If a patient misses more than one scheduled appointment, it may mean that catastrophic thoughts may be returning. Though a bit embarrassed, most are willing to tell you and to continue to work toward control of their anxiety.

CONCLUSION

This chapter provides guidelines for treating the panic patient. The three principal techniques recommended were changing attribution, *in vivo* desensitization, and biofeedback. At this point, note well this *caveat*. Two common strategies, useful for patients with generalized anxiety, do not work at all for these patients. The first is reassurance—"it will work out OK"—or—"We've had other patients just like you who have done OK." The second is testimonials. "I've treated a lot of patients who were afraid they were allergic to the anesthetic and have found that by controlling the fear, the physical reactions simply fade away." To this, one of our patients responded simply, "Different body!"

QUESTIONS AND EXERCISES

1. Two conceptual models were presented that relate one's thoughts to their fears or emotional responses. Explain the differences between these two models. What are their similarities? Identify an example which illustrates each of these two conceptualizations.

2. Identify a patient who has some fear or anxiety of dentistry. Interview this patient to determine how his or her cognitive activity contributes to the felt apprehension. Which of the two models applies? Determine ahead of time how you would present this information to the patient as an explanation for his or her response. Make a presentation to the patient and solicit the patient's feedback to see if your explanation appeared reasonably accurate to the patient. Devise and carry out a treatment plan for this patient's fear that is integrated within your dental treatment plan.

TEN

Treating Fearful Children

INTRODUCTION: DEFINING THE PROBLEM

Many dental health professionals are reluctant to treat children because they may be difficult to manage. Lack of training and experience with children and the attitude that treating children may not be worth the effort may exacerbate the problem. Students and clinicians not experienced in treating children often are not confident of their ability. This itself may contribute to difficulties (Weinstein et al., 1981).

Although strategies delineated in the previous chapters can be effective for patients of all ages, we have added this chapter to discuss special considerations for children because the goals for treating this age group differ from the general treatment goals for adults. Studies by experts in the field of childhood and pain, such as Forgione and Clark (1974); Kleinknecht, Klepac, and Alexander (1973); Lautch (1971); and Shoben and Borland (1951), show that most people feel their dental fears began in childhood. Creating positive attitudes toward dental care in children is an effective strategy to shape positive attitudes toward dentistry in adults and as such is a major goal of all treatment for children. Altering phobias is much more difficult and expensive. Early dental experiences should occur with a minimum of physical and psychological trauma.

Clinicians as far back as the turn of the century were concerned about the child's fear of dentistry. In 1895, McElroy noted: "Although the operative dentistry may be perfect, the appointment is a failure if the child departs in tears." Just as standard restorative, endodontic, and orthodontic techniques have been modified to treat deciduous dentition, the need to alter patient management has also been recognized. In fact, dental practitioners have long realized that the behavior of the child is the most important factor affecting actual treatment. Without patient cooperation, all dental procedures become difficult. Moreover, there is now the realization that today's treatment of the child is useful in laying a foundation for future acceptance of dental treatment. The need for effective, humane behavior management of children is obvious.

This chapter on treating children could easily have been expanded into a book. It was written to be of practical use to students and clinicians treating children and stems from both our research and clinical experience. We begin by discussing the need for creating a safe environment for children and then discuss, in detail, a variety of topics: child and parent assessment procedures, procedures for preventive management of problems, introduction of the child to the office, the parent in the operatory controversy, and effective management in the operatory. Toward the end of the chapter the following topics are included: general principles, i.e., what to do and what not to do when interacting with children, the appropriate role of the assistant, special consideration for older children and teenagers, and a discussion of aversive techniques and alternatives. The use of pharmacologic adjuncts is not discussed. We refer the reader to our discussions of nitrous oxide and premedication in Chapter 3 and to texts in child management (for example, Ripa and Barenie's *Management of Dental Behavior in Children*, Littleton, Mass.: P.S.G. Publishers, 1979).

A SAFE ENVIRONMENT

Towards the end of providing humane treatment, we attempt to create an accepting, "safe" child-oriented environment, a place for the child to explore and learn. We simply desire the child to learn that the dental office is not scary and that he or she has the opportunity to learn to cope with dental procedures. In doing so we recognize that children and adults are different and that developmental factors are at work. For example, young children have difficulty separating from their parents in a strange environment, and that while adults tend not to exhibit their fears, children have far fewer inhibitions.

Most children seen in the dental office are cooperative and allow the staff to function effectively and efficiently. As a result of long-term water fluoridation, children are less likely to need frequent restorative care; without traumatic restorative care, children are not as likely to misbehave. Of the minority who do misbehave, few present problems that are serious enough to disrupt treatment. Most misbehavior, such as whining or crying, is merely irritating. Although patience and the ability to "wait it out" are required of the practitioner, the child eventually comes to realize that his behavior will not produce its intended result and that other behaviors are more productive. Other misbehaviors, such as passive refusal to "open wide" or shouts of "I won't" or "I don't want to," or hypermotility—inability to sit still for more than a minute or so—can disrupt efficient treatment. The child who throws a tantrum—screams and flails legs and arms—not only disrupts treatment but endangers patient and staff well-being. Although procedures to manage disruptive and dangerous child behavior exist, measures taken to prevent such extreme behavior from emerging from existing anxiety or fear are well worth the effort.

Early in this chapter we focus on some techniques that you can use when working with children to *prevent* problems from developing or becoming unmanageable. Later in this chapter we will discuss management of these problems.

Survey of Child Management Problems

Weinstein et al. (1981) reported the results of surveying 145 Washington State general practitioners. An average of one-third of all patients seen per week (21/60) were children. Of that number, 6.5 percent presented difficulties. Fifteen percent of the practitioners reported 20 percent or more of child patients as problematic. Infants and toddlers were the most difficult age group to manage. Rates of successful treatment for problem categories were as follows: inability to communicate (29 percent), lack of cooperation (50 percent), "out-of-control behavior" (61 percent), and fear and anxiety (75 percent).

Techniques used to manage difficult children ranged from hand-over-mouth, mouth props, premedication with N_2O and Valium® to praise, desensitization, and careful explanation. No one technique was utilized by general practitioners significantly more often than other techniques or was more successful than any other. Pharmacological approaches were used in 26 percent of the difficult cases that were reported. These approaches were reported to be no more successful than non-drug approaches.

ASSESSMENT PROCEDURES

Questionnaires

Prior to discussing prevention, it is necessary to talk about assessment. Assessment should take place as early as possible, and information about parent and child is worth gathering. The parent in the reception room is often a source of information that can help you to better manage the child. Exactly what information should be sought is a function of your individual practice. However, we believe information that will help establish rapport and attune staff to possible behavior problems is extremely valuable. The following questions may be helpful:

1. Does the child have any pets, hobbies, special interests, or recent accomplishments?
   Yes   No
   If "yes," please list and/or give kind of pet and names.

2. Does the child have a nickname he enjoys?
   Yes   No
   If "yes," what is it?

3. Name of school, Grade.

4. Other children in family?
   Yes   No
   Please give name, age, and sex of each.

5. Has the child had any unpleasant contact with physicians or dentists?
   Yes   No
   If "yes," please describe.

6. How do you think your child will react to dental treatment?
   Good   Fair   Poor   Don't know
   Please comment.

7. How fearful are you of having your dental work done?
   Not at all   A little fearful   Somewhat fearful   Very fearful

8. How would you rate your own anxiety or nervousness at this moment?

Good   Fair   Poor   Don't know

9. Has your child had behavior or learning problems at school?

Yes   No

Please describe problems.

10. Does your child express concern about aspects of his teeth or mouth, such as a chipped or crooked tooth, decayed tooth, gum boil, etc.?

Yes   No

If "yes," please specify.

Studies attempting to identify factors influencing children's behavior in the dental office, summarized in a scholarly review by G.Z. Wright in 1975, have pinpointed three major variables. (1) The pleasantness or unpleasantness of any previous medical experiences will affect a child's behavior during his first dental visit (Martin et al., 1977). The similarity between dentist and physician is immediately obvious—both are called doctor, wear white coats, and employ receptionists and auxiliaries who dress similarly. Fear, especially in children, is often generalized from one situation to another similar one. (2) In many studies (Johnson and Baldwin, 1968 and 1969; Wright and Alpern, 1971; Bailey et al., 1973), maternal anxiety was found to be related to children's behavioral problems. Very anxious mothers have been found to exert a negative influence on children of all ages. (3) The child's awareness of a dental problem also creates apprehension. This may manifest itself as uncooperative behavior in the dental chair (Wright, Alpern, and Leake, 1973). Remember the anecdote about Joan in Chapter 1?

Not all problems in managing children are fear-related. Some children, even at a young age, chronically exhibit disruptive behaviors. At one extreme is the *hyperactive* child, who seems to have no control over his behavior. The clinical condition is characterized by excessive and unpredictable behaviors, unawareness of consequences, inability to focus on and concentrate on a task, and poor performance in school. Though not hyperactive, some children with little internal or external control of their impulses appear to mimic hyperactive behavior. Both actual and pseudo-hyperactive children usually have had maladaptive patterns of attention with parents and demonstrate noncompliant behavior with other adults.

The following questionnaire, adapted from the work of Forehand and McMahon (1981), who provide therapy for children and their parents, provides information that can be used to help structure a brief discussion with parents. The behaviors receiving the top three ranks are likely to manifest themselves in the operatory.

A few other factors associated with child fear and its manifestations in the dental office are worth mentioning. Age of the child has been often associated with fear. Younger children generally show greater fear and less cooperation. Children under age 3 presented the greatest difficulty, as communication between child and practitioner is difficult.

Socioeconomic class and sex are also factors. Low socioeconomic (poor) children are apt to be more frightened than their more affluent playmates (Hawley et al., 1974; Wright, 1980). Moreover, boys show less fear than girls, a cultural or biological phenomenon.

Parent Behavior Checklist

Check the behaviors below that represent problem areas with your child. Then rank-order the behaviors you checked from the most frequent to the least frequent.

_____ 1. Whine

_____ 2. Physical negative (attacks another person)

_____ 3. Destructiveness (destroys, damages, or attempts to damage objects)

_____ 4. Smart talk (teases, makes fun of, or embarasses others)

_____ 5. Noncompliance (does not do what he or she is told to do)

_____ 6. Ignore (fails to answer)

_____ 7. Yell or scream

_____ 8. Demand attention

_____ 9. Temper tantrum

The Preappointment Letter

We have noted anxious mothers tend to have uncooperative children. Interestingly, researchers have found that when mothers attempt to reduce their children's anxieties, they paradoxically increase anxiety. Apparently many mothers (and fathers) do not know how to prepare their children for dental visits. One practical approach to this problem involves sending a preappointment letter to parents of new child patients. In a study published in 1973, Wright, Alpern, and Leake report success with a letter that read like this:

> Dear Mrs.————:
>
> I am writing you because I am pleased with the interest you are showing in your child's dental health by making an appointment for a dental examination. Children who have their first dental appointment when they are young are likely to have a favorable outlook toward dental care throughout life.
>
> At our first appointment we will examine your child's teeth and gums, and take any necessary X-rays. For most children this proves to be an interesting and even pleasant occasion. All of the people on our staff enjoy children and know how to work with them.
>
> Parents play a most important role in getting children started with a good attitude toward dental care, and your cooperation is much appreciated. One of the useful things that you can do is to be completely natural and easygoing when you tell your child about his appointment. This approach will enable him to view his appointment primarily as an opportunity to meet some new people who are interested in him and want to help him to stay healthy.

Good general health depends in large part upon the development of good habits, such as sensible eating and sleeping routines, exercise, recreation, and the like. Dental health also depends upon good habits, including proper tooth-brushing, regular visits for dental care, and avoidance of excessive sweets. We will have a chance to discuss these points further during your child's appointment.

Best wishes, and I look forward to seeing you.

You may desire to send a short questionnaire, similar to the 10-item version given earlier, which asks for information on the child's interests, etc., with the letter.

Observation Checklists

In addition to questionnaires, your own observations are very valuable. Lists of behaviors to watch out for are helpful in collecting information. At times, especially when the child has had a history of difficulty receiving dental treatment, we ask the parent to direct the child in a structured activity and observe the parent in guiding the child. For example, "Mom, would you help Susie put this puzzle together?" or "After you watch me demonstrate, could you show Susie how to brush her teeth?" In the latter example, we utilize an auxiliary to provide not only instruction, but an assessment of how the mother functions. Note, occasionally a parent will be reluctant to interact with their child while being observed. Assure the parent that you understand, but want to see how the child interacts in this stressful, atypical dental setting.

We carefully observe parent and child not only in the waiting and treatment rooms but also during subsequent pre-visit activities and prophylaxis. Assessment is continuous. Chart notes always mention child and parent behavior and serve as a guide to future management. For example, the notation that the child cried during prophylaxis and asked repeatedly whether she would receive a "shot" is extremely helpful in developing an approach to the child for restorative treatment. Not knowing this information would be disastrous.

The following checklist may be a part of a comprehensive assessment:

BRIEF CHECKLIST FOR WAITING ROOM:

1. Is child upset, neutral, unhappy?
2. Does child leave sight of parent (to explore, play, etc.)?
3. Does mom scold, threaten, or otherwise coerce child?
4. Does mom ignore or pay minimal attention to child, even when upset?

PREVENTIVE STEPS WORTH TAKING FOR EVERY CHILD

Establish Rapport and Communicate Effectively

Establishing rapport, one of the foremost objectives when treating children, is not a "technique" that is applied for a few minutes at the beginning of each appointment. Rather, it is the recognition of each child as a unique individual. Although it is sometimes tempting to act as if children are a different species from adults, current research indicates they are not!

Rapport-building phrases such as, "Did you remember to bring your teeth today?" can be helpful, especially with younger children. With older children, their clothes, particularly the "billboard" tee-shirts, may give you clues to their interests. Taking a little time to learn about the child (including nickname, pets, hobbies, etc.), tells the child he or she is cared for. On the other hand, your own unique way of responding to adults with whom you are comfortable is also the appropriate way to respond to children in establishing and maintaining rapport. The difference is you use simpler concepts and vocabulary with children—without talking down to them. Children should be talked to at their level of comprehension. That means avoiding baby talk: employ words that have meaning for the patient. Development of your own word substitutes for foreign (to children) dental terminology can be useful; for example, rubber dam becomes rubber raincoat, and cotton roll, a tooth pillow, and a saliva ejector becomes a thirsty straw. The avoidance of scary words such as drill, shot, pain, and the use of lay terms ("this will feel like a little pinch") will make difficult procedures more acceptable. Practice this as if it were a second language. Everyone in an office should attempt to use the same terminology.

There are many ways to break the ice with children. Questions about their clothing, activities, and pets are commonly used. Whatever the tactic for initiating a conversation, you should plan to use open-ended questions that cannot be responded to in a simple "yes" or "no" fashion. For example, do not ask whether the child has a pet—ask him to tell you all about his pets.

Nonverbal communication is also important in establishing rapport. Touching or patting a child's shoulder communicates warmth; smiles convey approval and acceptance. Eye contact is important—when talking to children place yourself at the child's eye level. There is probably some truth in the clinical lore which states that children who avoid eye contact are not ready to cooperate fully. One very common mistake involves the assumption that all children of a particular chronological age think and feel the same. Though developmental trends permit some generalizations among children of the same chronological age, there is considerable variation in social and mental development.

INTRODUCTION OF THE CHILD TO THE OFFICE

The genesis of much fear-related behavior in the dental office lies in the poor early exposure to dentistry. As suggested in Chapters 1 and 2, such harmful initiation may be *direct*, a result of stressful dental treatment, or it may be *indirect*, a result of frightening comments and anxiety of other children and adults.

Feeling trapped and vulnerable contributes to fear. Therefore, *allow the child some control.* While parents and dentists need to be in control, it is probably best for children to allow them to exercise some control over events imposed upon them. Children allowed to *feel* in control show less fear. It is not difficult to structure simple choices for children. "Would you

268

like to begin (cleaning) here or there?" "I have banana and strawberry (fluoride), which would you like?" When allowing the child to decide, you must always follow through. Therefore, do not ask whether or not the child wants to have dental treatment.

Signal mechanisms may present an additional possibility: "Just raise your hand like this (dentist raises the appropriate hand in the desired manner) if anything bothers you." Although prompt verbal recognition of the signal is important, the dentist need not stop immediately. Kruper (1970) showed that an experimental mechanical signaling device, which allowed the child to inform the dentist when he was feeling discomfort, resulted in more cooperative behavior than children who did not have the device. It is interesting to note that such mechanical signaling devices may result in more cooperation but may not decrease child arousal (Corah, 1973). Mirrors, especially large hand mirrors, offer additional control in being able to see what is going on that some children relish.

Mismanagement may exacerbate existing developmental problems. For example, separation of a protesting three-year-old from his mother and not allowing the children any control over any events are both management techniques that enhance fear and related behavior.

Much has been written about introducing children to dental treatment. Usually, there has been considerable emphasis on reassurance and explanation. These techniques have limited utility, especially for highly anxious children (Howitt and Stricker, 1977).

Pre-exposing children to a pleasant, low stress dental experience was first reported in the early 1960s. Rosengarten (1961) brought children in for a pre-visit. During this time the office was introduced; treatment was provided on subsequent appointments. He found that children from ages 3–4.5 years benefited, those 5–5.5 did not. A few years later Laufer et al. (1964) used a similar technique with 6- to 7-year-old girls and found that the pre-visit significantly reduced fear.

Machen and Johnson (1974) compared two types of pre-visit intervention to a control condition. Preschool children with carious lesions were assigned to a control, desensitization, or modeling condition. After assignment to treatment groups, the experimental groups received the appropriate intervention one week prior to two restorative appointments. In the desensitization condition, procedures producing the least anxiety were presented first, followed by procedures that evoke more and more anxiety. The items related to these procedures and their order of presentation, from least to most "anxiety evoking" were as follows:

1. Prophylaxis contra-angle and pumice
2. Mirror and explorer
3. Rubber dam clamp
4. Rubber dam
5. Copalite
6. X-ray film
7. Handpiece
8. Anesthetic syringe
9. Dental operatory:
   a. Chair
   b. Light
   c. Water and air syringes
   d. Handpiece

The researchers noted that since the operatory itself is a high-anxiety stimulus, the intervention, until near the end of the session, was held in an ordinary room. The modeling condition consisted of viewing an 11-minute videotape of a child showing positive behavior during dental treatment and being reinforced by the dentist. Results of this study indicated that both experimental groups had similar positive behavior during subsequent restorative treatment.

Overall, we believe the experimental evidence supports the utilization of pre-visits for children who, because of existing caries or caries susceptibility, are likely to face stressful dental procedures. Those children who do not have caries or have a low caries susceptibility probably do not need such preparation, as dentistry for these children is not likely to be traumatic (Sawtell et al., 1974; Rouleau et al., 1981).

For children with no previous dental experience, we recommend that those between ages 3 and 5 be carefully introduced to the dental environment. The comforting behaviors of the dentist and his or her staff are critical. For example, Sawtell et al. (1974) found a friendly assistant to be as effective as desensitization and other treatments. Clearly, the accomplishment of dental procedures is secondary. Allowing the child to play while waiting in the dental office is a widely accepted pedodontic practice. A few pieces of child-size furniture and toys are all that are necessary. Play communicates to the child that the people that work here are child oriented.

We believe, from our experience, that the behavior of the dentist and staff in the waiting room will set the tone for the initial and subsequent visits. The following sequence of rapport-building behaviors is recommended for preschool children:

1. Greet child and parent, child first, in the waiting room shortly after their arrival. Talk to child for a short time. The "patter" will vary according to inclination and experience. We like to find a way to compliment the child, e.g., "I like your purple Star Wars shoes; they are neat!" And encourage a friendly dialogue, e.g., "Mom just got them for me. . . ." All sorts of interactions about clothing and movies are now possible. Pets and animals, e.g., "Tell me about your pets?" or "What animals do you like?" Sesame Street and holidays and birthdays are other ice breakers. When children are timid and do not respond, do not give up. Tell a brief story about something, e.g., "We have a dog named Josh. He is white with a curly tail and he likes children. This is his picture. Would you like to play with him?"

2. Introduce child to toys and tell him you will come back soon and show him some other "neat stuff."

3. Return and structure a choice for the child, while you take his hand, say "Now would you like to play with my special chair, or hold my special light (or brush or mirror)?"

4. If the child is very tentative, invite the parent to come in with you: "Mom, would you like to play with us too?" Most times, avoiding the trauma of separating child from parent is warranted. Moreover, parents can be very helpful if they are properly oriented to the role they will play. On the other hand, whether or not to allow the parent in the operatory is controversial.

Parent in the Operatory?

This is a long-standing controversy, with strong feelings on both sides. A large proportion of dentists treating children discourage the parents' presence in the operatory (Roder et al., 1961; Association of Pedodontic Diplomates, 1972 and 1981). Those who advocate keeping parents out argue that parents' presence disrupts procedures and provides an opportunity to communicate parental anxiety to the child. Those who advocate the parents' presence in the operatory suggest the positive influence of the parent in increasing the security and coping of the young child in an unfamiliar environment. A number of non-dental studies support this position. The research conducted in the dental environment is limited and inconclusive. Two studies of prophylaxis, one assessing physiological responses (Lewis and Law, 1958) and two assessing behavior (Allen and Evans, 1968) found no difference in children's responses. Similarly, Venham (1971) found no difference in the child's response to a series of two dental treatment visits, one with mother present and one without her presence. Frankl et al. (1962) found greater cooperative behavior during examination and subsequent treatment with mother present. On the other hand, Croxton (1967) reported that of 28 children referred to his private practice because they had exhibited behavior problems at other dental offices, most had had treatment while a parent was present. As part of his treatment, he excluded parents and reported, by the final visit, a 93 percent success rate.

An interesting non-dental study by Shaw and Routh (1981) with a small number of children sheds additional light on this controversy. Eigh-

272

teen-month and five-year-old children received routine immunizations in a pediatrician's office with and without the mother present. Comparisons between conditions indicate that behavior of children of both ages was more negative when mother was present. When mother was present, children cried longer after injections and continued to "fuss" more while being dressed and taken from the examination room. The findings were interpreted to mean that, given a stressful experience, children may inhibit protest if mother is absent.

It is clear that parents should not be routinely excluded from the operatory. There are a number of situations where parents can enhance management and reduce fears. Young children are prone to a number of fears, including fear of the unknown, separation from parents, and abandonment. Children commonly show such behavior up to about age 4. Children who cling to their parents and do not respond to an attractive play environment and overtures by dentist and assistant to enter the operatory, should not be forced to enter the operatory alone. On the other hand, depending on the goals of the visit, it may be useful to have the child inhibit his protestation.

It is useful to try to determine how the mother will behave in the operatory. Venham (1979) notes four broad categories of mothers. One group sat passively and remained uninvolved. A second group attempted to obtain cooperative behavior with no attempt to reduce anxiety and fear. These mothers used a variety of approaches, including comments, threats, and physical intervention. A third group focused the child's feelings and attempts to reduce upset through verbal reassurance and physical contact. A fourth group tried to both reduce upset and gain cooperation. Clearly, parental effectiveness varies. Many dentists provide instruction to parents on their role in the operatory; observation of the parent and child and determination of the parent's anxiety level are useful in the decision of whether or not the parent will be helpful or detrimental.

5. Structure additional chores for the child: "Would you like to climb into the chair from side (right side) or from here (left side)?"

6. Introduce everything. The "tell-show-do" approach, popularized by Addelston (1959), is extremely useful during initial appointments and in introducing completely new procedures during subsequent appointments. The approach is extremely simple. First *tell* the child about each new procedure and what is going to be done in it. The initial oral exam may proceed as follows: "We are going to count your teeth with our tooth counter." *Show* the child the instruments and describe any sensation that might be felt in positive or neutral terms. "This (mirror) is my counter. I will gently touch each tooth as I count." If the child is at all tentative, demonstrate: "Let's count your fingers with the counter." Similarly, the child's fingernail may be "cleaned" to introduce the sight, sound, and vibration of the handpiece prior to prophylaxis. "Now, did you bring your teeth today?" At this point, *do* what you said would be done: "I see you have lots of pretty teeth. Let's count. . . ." in using this approach, special care should be taken to use language and concepts the child can understand.

7. Use lots of praise (positive reinforcement) for any and all child cooperation. Always complete the visit on a positive note. Help the child feel a sense of accomplishment. Point out that he did a good job and thank him.

Many dentists give children a small gift after treatment. The gift is provided regardless of the behavior of the child. Though the behavioral literature indicates that such reinforcement should be provided contingent on appropriate behavior, it is our impression that the gift serves a useful function—it is a signal of acceptance of the child himself. Shapiro (1967) has suggested the possibility that a gift prior to the appointment may be more meaningful and helpful than a gift provided after the visit, and he has reported favorable reponses of children to his pre-operative gift. We think Dr. Shapiro has a good idea.

Another good idea may be the "contingent" use of stories played through headphones. Nash et al. (1984) found that when story tapes were interrupted following uncooperative behavior and resumed when the child cooperated, behavior fear was lower and cooperation was higher than in distraction (non-contingent use of story tapes) and control conditions.

The modeling management strategy, utilized by Machen and Johnson (1974), deserves elaboration because it may be utilized in conjunction with other management approaches. Allowing the child to observe another patient undergoing treatment is based on the assumption that information about what to expect and how to behave contributes to the reduction of fear and subsequent behavior problems.

The most critical factor determining the effectiveness of the modeling procedure is that the person perceives the model as similar to himself. In other words, a 7-year-old boy watching a 13-year-old girl would have little effect. It may be helpful if the model is perceived as somewhat fearful but able to overcome his fears and cope adequately. If a model is perceived to be confident and masterful, he is less likely to influence the observer—"He may not be afraid, but I am."

Many practitioners have long used modeling strategies by letting the younger child watch "big sister" through the appointment if they perceive a positive relationship between a confident sibling and the fearful child. A simple variation of the same strategy involves scheduling an unrelated fearful child to watch another child patient during his appointment.

A more complex use of the strategy involving both the tell-show-do technique and modeling, but which can be successfully used by the practitioner, was described in 1971 by pedodontist Papermaster:

> A "leader" child, who has had dental work done previously, is seated in the dental chair. One of the new patients is asked to assist in making the dental examination. He is given the mouth mirror and (a blunted) explorer. . . . Assist the child by holding his hand as he examines the teeth with the mouth mirror, checking the cavities and the fillings. He is then given the handpiece and is guided while one or two of the anterior teeth are polished with a rubber cup. He is given a pair of tweezers holding a piece of cotton and is asked to wipe off any particles on the teeth. The patient who has helped in the examination is then placed in the chair and another youngster is asked to help

in the examination, and so on until all the children have been examined. Fillings are done for those who have previously visited the office, and the children are dismissed. After one or two Saturday morning appointments, these children can be taken care of at any time during the week in the same manner as any adult.

Techniques discussed in this section are useful, not only for children, but also for fearful adults. Slow and careful introduction of fearful adults to the dental environment, tell-show-do, modeling, allowing supportive friends and family into the operatory, the importance of rapport and communication, and allowing some patient control are techniques that we recommend for *all* fearful patients. Melamed (1979), who has conducted a series of studies of modeling, presents a thorough review of this literature.

EFFECTIVE MANAGEMENT OF CHILDREN IN THE OPERATORY

The Guidance-Cooperation Model: A Useful Framework for Interaction with Children

An overall model of the practitioner-child interaction may be useful in conceptualizing your role and guiding your selection of child management strategies. The following model is derived from the work of two researchers whose contributions have broad application to all health care fields. In an article published in 1956, Szasz and Hollender distinguished three distinct models of doctor-patient relationships: the active-passive, guidance-cooperation and mutual participation models.

We believe the dental practitioner-child relationship is best characterized as "guidance-cooperation." In this model the patient is not completely passive, as is the case in surgery where general anesthesia is required (the active-passive model). Neither is the child permitted to participate with the practitioner in decisions concerning the dental procedure to be employed (the mutual participation model). In a treatment situation characterized by guidance-cooperation, the child is expected to look up to and obey the practitioner. This model has its prototype in the relationship of parent and child and is especially relevant for pedodontics where the practitioner is in a helping relationship with a young child. Research conducted in 1978 at the University of Washington School of Dentistry Pedodontics Clinic has indicated that the use of "directive guidance"—a straightforward assertive statement of expectation with feedback concerning the child's behavior—led to cooperative child behavior. For example: "Open a little wider, please—Good boy!" On the other hand, permissive behavior, such as saying, "Are you ready for me to begin now? Pretty please?" and coercive behavior, such as threats of scolding, resulted in substantial resistant and uncooperative child behavior (Wurster, Weinstein, and Cohen, 1979).

A Study of Child Management

Subsequently, we undertook a major study of how children are managed in community dental offices. The major goal of the study was to identify effective and ineffective patterns of interaction between dentist and child and assistant and child. Twenty-five dentists volunteered. Fifty regular child patients of those dentists participated. Dentists identified 3- to 5-year-old children in their practices. These children were then screened by the dentist during their next appointment. At that time, child behavior during prophylaxis was observed and dental health was recorded. Children in need of treatment requiring two or more sessions in which injections would be required were eligible for participation in the study.

Dentists agreed to not use nitrous oxide or any other premedication. Aside from this prohibition, they were asked to treat the child as they ordinarily would. All sessions were videotaped by an experienced technician. Seventy-two usable videotapes from 23 offices have been analyzed (Weinstein et al., 1982).

A reliable but complex coding scheme was developed to help us analyze the data. Dimensions of child behavior included Movement and Physical Positioning, Verbal Behavior, and Comfort. Behaviors within these dimensions, for example, crying, discomfort, and inappropriate movement were combined into fear and non-fear-related categories. Dentist and assistant dimensions included various forms of guidance—directs, explains, sets rules, coaxes, empathizes, i.e., questions about feelings, reassure, etc.; physical control and verbalization, i.e., silence, dental to child, distraction, etc.

To identify patterns of interaction between dentist and child and assistant and child, probabilities that child fear-related behavior *followed* both dentist and assistant behavior were determined. This was done for each procedure and for the appointment as a whole. Needless to say, the analysis was complex and required the use of a computer. On the other hand, the results were very easy to understand. We will discuss the most important results, one dimension at a time. First for the dentist, next for the assistant.

EFFECTS OF DENTIST BEHAVIOR

When the dentist used directive guidance, fear-related behaviors were lowest after the use of direction and reinforcement. Specific feedback resulted in less fear-related behavior than general feedback. Direction was more effective than rules, which are general directions used beforehand in anticipation of problem behavior, and rhetorical questions, e.g. "Could you open your mouth?" Young children respond to a rhetorical question as if it were a real question and not a social convention. Specific reinforcement, e.g., "I like the way you keep your mouth open," more effective than general reinforcement, i.e., "Good boy."

These findings clearly support learning theory, which states that the immediacy and strength of both discriminative stimuli (cues) and reinforcement (feedback) are important in understanding and controlling the behavior of the organism in the environment. Therefore, it was not surprising to find that the use of rhetorical questions, such as "Would you like to get into the chair now?" (which are less immediate and strong), were much less effective in decreasing fear-related behaviors than specific direction.

Explanation was not the most effective technique with young children. Only during the low-stress chair placement phase did the use of explanation precede a significant decrease in fear-related behaviors. Some support for this finding is found in Howitt and Stricker's (1965) work, which determined that "clarification" (explanation) was more effective with mildly anxious than highly anxious children. Evidence also exists that information about anticipated events, such as surgery, may not decrease anxiety. Explanation is not a panacea. Three- to 5-year-old fearful children usually are not helped in fearful situations by rational discussion. In fact, it is our clinical impression that fearful children sometimes question and encourage explanation to avoid anticipated dental procedures.

Coercion and coaxing both are ineffectual management procedures. Dentists seem to use these procedures when they are frustrated by the child. Often the dentist's voice indicates his or her frustration, which may further exacerbate the situation. Emotional reactions are usually reciprocal: the child's fear-related behavior (stimulus) uses the dentist's frustration (response), which in turn causes further fear-related behavior in the child (stimulus). We hypothesize that by the time the dentist resorts to coercion and coaxing, he or she has already lost control of the situation.

In addition, the ability of preschool children to inhibit their own behaviors on demand is somewhat limited. Guidance to do something is usually more successful than a message to stop or slow down a behavior. Clinicians, therefore, should focus on what the child is to do. Inhibiting ongoing behavior is especially problematic for young children. It is better to prevent the problems before they emerge.

Questioning for feeling, which attempts to elicit and recognize the child's feelings, appears to be the most effective empathic behavior. Reassurance, which may deny or ignore feelings, such as "Everything will be okay, don't worry," is followed by a greater probability of fear-related behavior. Reassurance, as Bernstein and associates (1974) have noted, does not really reassure. "Analysis of dentists' empathy responses shows that reassurances were used most frequently during injection, rubber dam, and drilling phases, with very few occurrences recorded in earlier phases. Reassurances are used most frequently in stressful situations and have little effect in reducing fear.

279

These results support the position of Rogers (1961) who has long held that emphatic understanding—a combination of listening for another's feelings and expressing concern for those feelings—is a critical ingredient in helping relationships. Understanding makes the dentist aware of the patient's perception of dental procedures. In turn, the patient is more willing to trust the clinician, which influences how the patient structures the situation psychologically and how he subsequently responds.

Put-downs and ignoring/denying fear-related behaviors are ineffective and should be avoided. Interestingly, such behaviors resulted in a pattern similar to that found in extinction curves; when reinforcement is withheld, behavior does not dramatically decrease but decreases slowly. Such dentist behaviors may contribute to the etiology of phobias (see Chapter 2).

Other studies indicate patting the child, a warm nonverbal gesture, is useful in reducing fear-related behavior in young children. And child management procedures such as directing, explaining, reinforcing, distracting, or reassuring are more effective when the dentist is in working contact with the child. Stopping dental procedures to manage child behavior is less effective. In such situations, halting treatment may inadvertently reinforce the child's fear-related behaviors. That is, the child is being rewarded for fear-related behaviors by the dentist's stopping the treatment.

Distracting young children does not appear to be an extremely useful approach. It is especially poor during the rubber dam application. After an injection, children are generally wary. Distraction at that time may be perceived as a cue that another stressful procedure lies ahead.

In all, the evidence suggests that providing immediate direction and specific reinforcement are most consistently followed by a reduction in the child's fear-related behaviors. Patting and stroking behaviors also tend to be followed by a lessening of fear behaviors. Questioning for feeling is a useful technique: ignoring or denying child's feelings is not. Reassurance is surprisingly ineffectual. Coercion, coaxing, and put-downs tend to be followed by a substantial increase in fear-related responses by the child. Explanations, although frequently used, do not appear to significantly reduce fear-related responses. Moreover, stopping treatment *during treatment* to manage the child appears to result in more fear-related behaviors.

GENERAL PRINCIPLES OF CHILD MANAGEMENT

A number of general principles emerge from our work and that of our colleagues who study child management.

The Positive "What To Do"

USE SPECIFIC DIRECTION GIVING. Use direct and specific requests for cooperation: "Please open your mouth, now"; "Turn this way; open a little wider"; "Put your hands back into your lap." Give the child the directions throughout the appointment and let him know what you expect him to do and not to do, i.e, "Keep your hands on your lap until I tell you it's O.K. to move again," or "Keep your head still, please, until I finish with this part."

PRAISE ALL COOPERATIVE BEHAVIORS. You cannot praise or "stroke" the child too frequently. When the child makes any attempt to respond to a directive, for example, "open wide," praise him. Most importantly, do not forget to praise him when he is sitting still and cooperating. Much too often, we do not pay attention to the child until his behavior causes problems.

USE SPECIFIC REINFORCEMENT. Specific reinforcement consists of expressing positive feelings to the patient for his cooperation, and explaining *exactly* what the patient did that the dentist found helpful. This technique is one of the single most effective procedures you can use to elicit cooperation. All of us, particularly children, like to know when we "do good."

"It really helps when you hold so still. . . . Good helping."

"You follow my directions very well, I appreciate that."

"Holding your head like that helps me get done much faster!"

"I like it when you hold your mouth open so wide. You make it easy for me."

THINK OF NEW AND CREATIVE WAYS TO PRAISE SPECIFIC BEHAVIOR. General reinforcement consists of an expression of positive feelings to the patient for cooperation which does not specify a particular behavior. For example:

"You are a great patient."

"You're doing just fine."

"Good patient."

"That-a-girl."

Everyone likes to receive some general reinforcement occasionally. However, it is not nearly as effective as the use of specific reinforcement in obtaining cooperation from a patient because they can only guess at what they are doing that pleases you.

EXPRESS YOUR CONCERN FOR THE CHILD. Ask the child how he is feeling or if he is comfortable. Demonstration of your concern for the child is important to him. Verbal demonstration, e.g., "Are you okay?" "Is it too tight?" and signal mechanisms, e.g., "I want you to raise your hand if something is bothering you," are excellent management practices. Dentist patting, a comforting gesture, is often appreciated.

KEEP YOUR COOL. To show anger in response to a child's behavior will only make matters worse. If you can ignore irritating but non-interfering behavior such as crying or whining, do so. If you cannot, do not retaliate with coercion. We are not saying you should not show your displeasure. A statement like, "I get mad (or unhappy, etc.) when you . . . ," when said in a calm voice, is more likely to succeed than coercion or permissiveness.

USE VOICE CONTROL. Frequently a sudden change in tone or volume can be used to gain the attention of a child who is not cooperating. What is said is not critical; it is the change of voice that gains the attention of the child. Return to the previous tone or volume as soon as the child begins to respond to your voice change. Again, do not show anger.

ALLOW THE CHILD TO PLAY A ROLE. Structure choices for the child to make. For example, "Shall we count the top or bottom teeth first?" "Would you like me to help you into the chair or would you like to climb up yourself?" Most children want to be as adult as possible and enjoy the role of "helper." Helpers hold mirrors, swabs, etc., and receive praise for the good work they do. This is especially useful for preschoolers.

STRUCTURE TIME. Specifying the amount of time that the child will spend in the chair may be useful, as it allows the fearful patient to pace himself. Knowledge that discomfort will be only for three minutes, or that only one minute is left before a procedure ends or a break occurs can be very helpful. We also show children an egg timer and negotiate in-chair time, after which the child will be able to play with toys in the waiting room while the dentist goes off and performs other duties.

USE POSITIVE SUGGESTIONS. The role of suggestion (describing and predicting future events) in effective patient management is an important but almost totally unresearched topic. Neilburger (1978) presents the only clinical investigation. He compared the effect of suggestion ("When I brush your teeth it will tickle and make you laugh even more. You don't have to laugh too much, but many children do.") to no suggestion ("Hello, Billy. How are you? Today we are going to clean your teeth with a magic toothbrush and toothpaste."). Results indicated that suggestion decreased resistant behaviors. The most positive reaction was found among the six- to eight-year-old children.

The Negative: What to Avoid

AVOID COERCION, BELITTLEMENT, AND PERMISSIVE-NESS. All are really very similar. They indicate to the child that you are ineffective in managing their behavior. They make things worse.

AVOID ELABORATE EXPLANATIONS. This is not important especially after you have begun the treatment. Do not try to talk a child into cooperation. Explain while you work, do not stop to explain, and do not get caught up in responding to a barrage of questions. Tell the child you will respond to questions after the treatment and live up to your promise.

DO NOT RELY HEAVILY ON RULE-SETTING OR DISTRAC-TION. Both have limited effectiveness. Distraction probably should not be used after the initial injection. Children learn quickly.

AVOID PREMATURE REASSURANCE. "It's going to be O.K.," "It won't bother you for very long," "There, that wasn't so bad," "Almost done, just a little longer," are at best, overused. They tend to be ineffective. When a child protests, you can express empathy and understanding by saying something like, "I know you don't really want to be here," (or "like this part"), or "I wish you didn't have to do this too," *but* "When you are at the dentist's, there are lots of funny things you have to do that you don't do anywhere else. So let's get on with it and finish. Then we can go and do something else." Then in a firm, but calm voice, continue with a specific direction or command.

EFFECTS OF ASSISTANT BEHAVIOR

Now we will present some results of our work that have implications for the role of the assistant in child management (Weinstein et al., 1983). Gently holding the child *prior* to disruptive movement and restraining appears to be well-accepted and effective assistant behaviors in management of difficult children. Other behaviors, e.g., reinforcement of positive behavior, and questioning for feeling appear to be used by assistants with some effectiveness. Surprisingly, assistant pats were ineffective. This may be because pats are given only when the child is already showing fear and are not used in prevention.

Other factors that influence assistant behavior have also been explored. Though the correlations were only moderate between assistant and dentist behaviors, the additional analysis of patterns of behavior reveal assistants look to dentists to model behavior. Unfortunately, dentist control of the situation, though essential, has caused auxiliaries to play less than optimal roles. We agree with Starkey (1975) that "the dental auxiliary must understand, accept and share the philosophy of the dentist; otherwise, she will be unable to support him. . . ." There is much to be gained by enhancing the assistant's support role in this area. Moreover, there may be a need for formal instruction in this area in dental assisting programs. At the very least, a structured in-service training or orientation program is indicated.

TREATING THE OLDER CHILD AND TEENAGER

Although most of what we have written focuses on the fear-related behaviors of the young child, older children and adolescents can be fearful. Fear in the older child often seems to center on the injection. Many of these children are old enough to travel to their appointments independently. No-shows are a frequent problem. With these children, age 10+, we usually expect too much. The natural tendency is to treat the physically mature child as if he were socially and mentally mature. In reality, the huge 12-year-old may have the emotional control of a 6-year-old, whereas a childlike wisp of a prepubescent teenager may show the mental maturity of a young adult.

Flexibility and frustration tolerance are therefore important for the clinician. We try, by trial and error, to communicate effectively. We are careful not to enter into the dynamics of any ongoing developmental difficulties. This means that we do *not* take on the parental role. We try to establish and maintain a personal relationship with these children that is independent of the parent. When they do not meet our expectations, e.g., they fail appointments or otherwise do not agree to work on their fears with us, we do not punish them, verbally or otherwise. Anger is counter-productive. These children are frequently yelled at by parents, teachers, and other adults. Their day is filled with coercion; their response is resistance, passive or otherwise.

We communicate with these children in an adult-to-adult manner. Rapport may be difficult to establish, as the child may not be responsive to our conversation. We encourage *all* verbalizations with those who are silent by giving lots and lots of positive verbal strokes for the most meager utterances. We try to show the child that we like him or her.

At an early point, we discuss with the child whether or not he or she desires to overcome his fears and to receive treatment. We present a treatment plan not only to the parent or parent and child but also to the child alone. We make it clear that he or she has decisional and behavioral control over all dental events and that we are working for *him* (or *her*), even though his parents are paying the freight. We will go at his speed.

Also, we tell him we recognize that coming here and facing his fears is work. He deserves to feel proud and be rewarded. A regular time is chosen for appointments. We recommend that parent, child, and dentist enter into a contractual agreement regarding attendance at sessions and completion of homework assignments, if needed. For example, we have negotiated an agreement, after two missed appointments with a sixteen-year-old, that mom provide us with five dollars per completed appointment to be provided to the child in the form of a much desired fishing reel after treatment is completed. Moreover, charges for missed appointments were to be paid for both by parent and the fund established to buy the reel.

If a parent expresses concern over "bribing" the child, it will be necessary to clarify the difference between bribery and reinforcement. A "bribe" is defined as something offered to induce dishonest acts. Reinforcement is used to teach appropriate behaviors; it is used temporarily because the behavior does not, at the time, have intrinsic reward.

AVERSIVE MANAGEMENT TECHNIQUES AND ALTERNATIVES

There is a class of child management procedure that causes children, and the authors, discomfort. These techniques are primarily oriented toward compliance and not management of fear. The techniques in this category include strapping the child down or wrapping him in a sheet and placing a hand over the mouth, and perhaps nose as well.

In a 1980 survey of attitudes and practices of members of the American Academy of Pedodontics, almost 98 percent of all members, including Diplomates, used "hand over mouth" in selected cases. Purposes noted included gaining cooperation and attention and "dampening vocal noise." Other restraints were used in selected cases by 86 percent of the members.

Our belief is that it is unfortunate that so many clinicians utilize some form of restraint when a positive management approach fails. Such action indicates low tolerance for children's demonstration of upset and fear and a procedure-oriented practice philosophy. We see a number of adults in our Fear Clinic who were abused by these techniques when they were children. When reaching adulthood, these individuals avoid dental care almost completely. Such procedures go a long way to perpetuate the negative stereotypes of dentists. *Both hand over mouth and other restraints should not be used in dental practice, except during an emergency.* The use of aversive techniques so that a prophylaxis or a restoration can be accomplished is not warranted. Few parents, if given a choice, would consent to such procedures. It is our bet that dentists who rely heavily on such procedures do so without the presence of parents in the operatory.

Hand-over-mouth technique has been used for over 50 years. Most advocates specify that the technique is a last resort, to be used to establish communication after all other approaches have failed and the child's behavior remains uncontrolled. Even advocates warn that the technique, which involves removing the clinician's hand from the child's mouth only when the child cooperates, is contra-indicated for children under age 3, those who are mentally impaired, and for children who have been sedated. Moreover, there are numerous other caveats, the most important

287

being that the clinician not behave emotionally and control his own response. This is most difficult; techniques of last resort are not readily employed without emotion, especially when the dentist is frustrated and angry. The scenario of a screaming, flailing child is emotionally charged. Children can sense the anger and inadequacy of the clinician and do not respond positively in such situations. A useful description of the technique is found in an article by Levitas (1974).

I place my hand over the child's mouth to muffle the noise. I bring my face close to his and talk directly into his ear. "If you want me to take my hand away, you must stop screaming and listen to me. I only want to talk to you and look at your teeth." After a few seconds, this is repeated, and I add, "Are you ready for me to remove my hand?" Almost invariably there is a nodding of the head. With a final word of caution to be quiet, the hand is removed.

As it leaves the face, there may be another wail with the garbled request, "I want my mommy." Immediately the hand is replaced. The admonition to stop screaming is repeated, and I add, "You want your mommy?" Once again the head bobs. And then I say, "All right, but you must be quiet, and I will bring her in as soon as I am finished. O.K.?" Again, the nod—and the hand is slowly lowered. My assistant is always present during HOME to help restrain flailing arms and legs so that no one is physically injured. By restraining the child he can be made aware of the fact that his undesirable coping strategies are not necessary or useful.

While the child is composing himself, I begin to talk—about his clothes, about his freckles, about his pets, about almost anything, and no reference is made to what has gone before. As far as I am concerned, that is done and over. If there is an attempt on the part of the child to start again, a gentle but firm reminder that the hand will be replaced is usually enough to make him reconsider. It is sometimes difficult to convey

HOME with the written word, for voice control and modulation are essential for HOME to be most effective.

There are variations of the hand-over-mouth technique. Lenchner and Wright (1975) note the importance of adequate preparation of the assistant; he or she must know his or her role, as use of this technique is rarely planned.

Alternative procedures do exist. We have found that aversive techniques are often used prematurely. Children do not show tantrum behavior in the chair without warning. They show numerous signs of fear and upset, which usually go ignored or are attended to by superficial reassurance. Often, adequate time is not taken to establish support and to reinforce positive behaviors. Moreover, there is usually a clinician desire to complete procedures within a given period of time. Stopping or not completing a procedure is viewed as a defeat and is intolerable to some. Ending a procedure when a child is getting tired or upset is a good idea. In doing so we close the appointment on a positive note and praise the child for whatever cooperation he has shown. In some circumstances, we have praised the child for just sitting in the chair.

When the child begins to panic, e.g., screaming and flailing, there is little that we can do to effectively manage his fear. It is too late. The child should be told that he has done well and that we are done for the day. The following appointment should have modest goals—considerable positive verbal reinforcement for any bit of cooperation, and play interspersed with treatment. The use of pharmacological agents such as chloral hydrate or nitrous oxide are distinct possibilities. The modeling of other siblings and friends is another alternative. Clearly, the parent must understand what is going on and be part of the decision-making. Treatment of this sort is more costly than hand-over-mouth, but worth the expense in the long run.

In all, a wide variety of child management procedures have been presented. For the child, the dental office may be an unfamiliar or threatening environment. Altering the child's perceptions, through careful introduction to dentistry, and attention to communication itself will yield cooperative children with minimal fear. In the long run, the preventive approach is most efficient.

CONCLUSION

Creating a safe atmosphere for children requires careful introduction of the child to the dental environment. As such, assessment procedures that point to the consequences of child and parent are valuable. Positive dentist management of the child involves minimizing coercion, coaxing, premature verbal reassurance, and other such behaviors, while maximizing direction, feedback, and emphatic behaviors such as questioning for feelings. While under-utilized in behavior management, a set of effective/ineffective behavior guidelines for assistants has been identified. When a positive approach fails, hand-over-mouth and other aversive procedures are not generally warranted. Alternative procedures exist.

QUESTIONS AND EXERCISES

1. Consider the preappointment letter. Can you think of any changes you would make in this to fit your own style and/or office practice? If so, draft such a letter.

2. Reflecting back to Chapter 2, on the origins of dental fear, consider how each of the child management strategies described here could serve to prevent the development of fear.

3. Develop a list of phrases that you can use in various situations, e.g., putting on the rubber dam, which (a) convey interest and empathy for children, (b) can serve to reinforce specific behaviors, and (c) give specific and clear directions that will be unambiguous for the child of different ages.

4. How can you give a child patient a sense of control? Give specific examples.

Appendices

Appendix A.
About the University of Washington Dental Fear Research Clinic

We thought that you would like to know something about the setting in which many of the clinical techniques described in this book were developed.

The University of Washington Dental Fear Research Clinic was established in 1981 by Drs. Milgrom and Weinstein and Mr. Getz. Its mission is to treat adult individuals who are fearful of dentistry to the degree that they are unwilling or unable to receive care anywhere else. It is a separate 4 chair clinic within the School and operates as an intramural faculty research oriented clinic. Patients are primarily self referred and learn of the clinic through coverage by the media of the clinic. Approximately 30–40 patients are seen during the 2 days the clinic is open each week.

The clinic also serves as a laboratory for research, a training facility for graduate research fellows, and a clinical setting for dental students and general practitioners enrolled in CDE courses. The clinic operates with a hygienist one day a week and an assistant for both days. Regular dental fees are charged for all work performed. Psychological treatment is in addition to basic dental treatment fees. Each new patient is evaluated by a clinic psychologist and is treated by a dentist-psychologist team. The clinic is self supporting.

The University is located in Seattle, Washington and has an enrollment of 34,000, making it the largest University on a single campus in the West. The School of Dentistry graduated its first class in 1952 and has an enrollment of about 300 students in dentistry, dental hygiene, and the biological and behavioral sciences. The city population is approximately 500,-000. The greater metropolitan area population is 1.2 million. State population is 4 million.

Appendix B.
Making a Referral to a Mental Health Specialist

Selecting a mental health professional to assist you in overcoming a patient's fear can be a difficult task. Professional approaches range from Freudian analysis to life style clarification. The therapeutic approach which has been proven most effective with specific fears and phobias is called behavioral or cognitive-behavioral therapy. It is broadly based upon the principles of learning, and desensitization. Once you have completed reading this book you will have a good idea of this approach and the kind of questions to ask a prospective referral.

The type of professional which most often works with this kind of individual using a behavior approach is a psychologist. A psychiatrist is an M.D. with psychological training. In general, they are either oriented toward psychodynamic therapy (Freudian) or specialize in treatment of psychiatrically disturbed individuals, and rely more frequently on various therapeutic drug regimens. This does not mean that we feel that psychologists are always the best qualified and most appropriate referral. There are many psychiatrists, therapists, and counselors competent to work with these kinds of problems. The guidelines presented here are provided only to outline a straightforward way to find assistance.

Consequently, if you do not have a personal contact, we recommend you first contact your state psychological association. They should be able to provide you the name of a clinical psychologist in your area specializing in the treatment of anxiety reactions and phobias. Because of the difficulty of making referrals with fearful patients, it has been our experience that establishing a relationship with a specific individual results in greater success.

Once you have a name, contact the individual by phone and discuss the situation and the reason for your call. It is helpful to be as specific as possible. Use the assessment process outlined in Chapter 4. Outline: 1) the patient's self report of his or her past dental experiences, 2) your behavioral observations of the patient, and 3) a tentative diagnosis of the patient's fear type. For example, "The patient last went to a dentist approximately 7 years ago and reports that all her previous experiences were terrifying. She shook noticeably during her initial exam and her pulse was in the high 90's. She appears to have a lot of generalized anxiety. She reports being a worrier and frequently has physical symptoms when she is upset. It appears that she is also afraid of flying, and perceives life in general as very stressful." It may also be helpful to describe how many hours of work you see necessary in order for you to restore the patient back to health and whether you have discussed the possibility of referral with the patient.

Finally, do not hesitate to question the psychological professional on his areas of client specialization and treatment approaches. Psychologists do not treat "anyone who walks in the door," and are as interested as you are in making appropriate matches between therapist and patient.

Appendix C. Treatment Modality Checklist

Treatment strategies are listed under those Diagnosis Categories where they are *most frequently* utilized. This, of course, does not mean certain strategies will or will not be used from every category with a particular patient.

Treatment Strategy	Primary control issues	
I. Fear of Specific Stimuli		
___ presentation of mind-body-pain model	behavioral	X
___ tell-show-do	cognitive	X
___ elaborate explanations of how and why	information	
___ in vivo desensitization	retrospective (cause/effect)	___
___ distraction		
___ relaxation, deep breathing, pain tolerance,		
homework		
II. Distrust of Dental Personnel		
___ Emphasis on patient decision making and choice; use	behavioral	X
of signal mechanisms; checks on patient status		
___ dentist initiated rest periods		
___ frequent social reinforcement	cognitive	___
___ two-way communication	information	___
___ *extra* rapport building prior/post treatment time by	retrospective	___
dentist		
___ patient "assertiveness" training		

Treatment Modality Checklist (*Continued*)

III. Generalized Anxiety

___ focus on cognitive coping skills used under stress (self-image) — behavioral — X

___ chronic avoider/procrastination behaviors—app. control — cognitive — |

___ compartmentalize dental from other problems; supportive therapy and bibliotherapy — information — |

___ cognitive control of anticipatory thoughts including — retrospective

___ homework

___ distraction

___ hypnosis

IV. Fear of Catastrophe

___ relaxation—control of bodily sensations: — behavioral — X

___ deep breathing/muscle relaxation — cognitive — |

___ hypnosis — information — |

___ presentation of mind-body model (a la Schacter) — retrospective

___ changing cognitions surrounding *specific event*

___ re-definition of "fear," and "success"

___ distraction

Bibliography

Accepted Dental Therapeutics 41st ed., Chicago: American Dental Association, September (1982).

Addelston, K.K. Child patient training. *Fortnightly Review of the Chicago Dental Society* 38:7–11 (1959).

Agras, S., Sylvester, D., and Oliveau, D. The epidemiology of common fears and phobia. *Comprehensive Psychiatry* 10:151–156 (1979).

Allen, B.P., and Evans, R.I. Video tape recording in social psychological research: an illustrative study of pedodontia. *Psychological Reports* 23:1115–1119 (1968).

Allen, W.A. In P. Sykes (Ed.), *Dental Sedation and Anesthesia.* London, SAAD, 1979.

Association of Pedodontic Diplomates. Survey of attitudes and practices in behavior management. *Pediatric Dentistry* 3:246–250 (1981).

Association of Pedodontic Diplomates. Technique for behavior management—A survey. *Journal of Dentistry for Children* 39:368–372 (1972).

Auerbach, S.M., Kendall, P.C., Cuttler, H.F., and Levitt, N.R. Anxiety, locus of control, type of preparatory information and adjustment to dental treatment. *Journal of Consulting and Clinical Psychology* 44:809–818 (1976).

Averell, J.R. Personal control over aversive stimuli and its relationship to stress. *Psychological Bulletin* 80:286–303 (1973).

Baab, D., and Weinstein, P. Oral hygiene instruction using a self-inspection index. *Community Dentistry and Oral Epidemiology* 11:174–179 (1983).

Babajews, A.V., and Ivanyi, L. The relationship between in vivo and in vitro reactivity of patients with a history of allergy to local anesthetics. *British Dental Journal* 152(11):385–7 (1982).

Bailey, P.M., Talbot, A., and Taylor, P.P. A comparison of maternal anxiety levels with anxiety levels manifested in the child dental patient. *Journal of Dentistry for Children* 45:62–67 (1978).

Bandura, A. Self-efficacy: toward a unified theory of behavioral change. *Psychological Review* 84:191–215 (1977).

Barash, D.P. Human ethology: displacement activities in a dental office. *Psychological Reports* 34:947–949 (1974).

Barber, T.X. Physiological effects of "hypnotic suggestions." A critical review of recent research (1960–64). *Psychological Bulletin* 63:201–222 (1965).

Barenie, J.T. Inhalation conscious sedation: Nitrous oxide analgesia. In L.W. Ripa and J.T. Barenie (Eds.), *Management of Dental Behavior in Children.* Littleton, Massachusetts: PSG Publishing Co., 1979.

Beck, A.T. *Cognitive Therapy and Emotional Disorders.* New York: New American Library, 1979.

Berger, D.E. Assessment of the analgesic effects of nitrous oxide on the primary dentition. *Journal of Dentistry for Children* 39:265–268 (1972).

Bernstein, D.A., and Kleinknecht, R.A. Multiple approaches to the reduction of dental fear. *Journal of Behavior Therapy and Experimental Psychology* 13:187–292 (1982).

Bernstein, D.A., Kleinknecht, R.A., and Alexander, L.D. Antecedents of dental fear. *Journal of Public Health Dentistry* 39:113–124 (1979).

Bernstein, L., Bernstein, R.S., and Dana, R.H. *Interviewing: A Guide for Health Professionals.* New York: Appleton-Century-Crofts, 1974.

Billings, A.G., and Moos, R.H. The role of coping responses and social resources in attenuating the stress of life events. *Journal of Behavioral Medicine* 4:139–157 (1981).

Bolles, R.C., and Fanselow, M.S. A perceptual-defensive-recuperative model of fear and pain. *The Behavioral and Brain Sciences* 3:291–323 (1980).

Borland, L.R. Odontophobia—inordinate fear of dental treatment. *Dental Clinics of North America* 6:683–395 (1962).

Brandon, R.K., and Kleinknecht, R.A. Fear assessment in a dental analogue setting. *Journal of Behavioral Assessment* 4:317–325 (1982).

Butler, J.H., Abbott, D.M., and Bush, F.M. Biofeedback as a method of controlling bruxism. *Journal of Dental Research* 55:B310 (1976).

Cannistraci, A.J. A method to control bruxism: biofeedback-assisted relaxation therapy. *Journal of the American Society for Preventive Dentistry* 6:12–15 (1976).

Cannon, W.B. *Bodily Changes in Pain, Hunger, Fear and Rage* (2nd ed.). New York: Appleton-Century-Crofts, 1929.

Carlsson, S.G., Gale, E.N., and Ohman, A. Treatment of temporomandibular joint syndrome with biofeedback training. *Journal of the American Dental Association* 91:602–605 (1975).

Chaves, J.F., and Brown, J.M. Self-generated strategies for the control of pain and stress. Paper presented at the annual meeting of the American Psychological Association, August 1978, Toronto, Canada.

Clum, G.A., Luscomb, R.L., and Scott, L. Relaxation training and cognitive redirection strategies in the treatment of acute pain. *Pain* 12:175–183 (1982).

Clum, G.A., Scott, L., and Burnside, J. Information and locus of control as factors in the outcome of surgery. *Psychological Reports* 45:867–873 (1979).

Connolly, J., Hallam, R.S., and Marks, I.M. Selective association of fainting with blood-injury-illness fear. *Behavior Therapy* 7:8–13 (1976).

Corah, N.L. Assessment of a dental anxiety scale. *Journal of Dental Research* 48:496 July-August (1969).

Corah, N.L. Effect of perceived control on stress reduction in pedodontic patients. *Journal for Dental Research* 52:1261–1264 (1973).

Corah, N.L. Relaxation and musical programming as a means of reducing psychological stress during dental procedures. *Journal of the American Dental Association* 103:232–234 (1981).

Corah, N.L., Gale, E.N., and Illig, S.J. Psychological stress reduction during dental procedures. *Journal of Dental Research* 58:1347–1351 (1979a).

Corah, N.L., Gale, E.N., and Illig, S.J. The use of relaxation and distraction to reduce psychological stress during dental procedures. *Journal of the American Dental Association* 98:388–394 (1979b).

Croxton, W.L. Child behavior and the dental experience. *Journal of Dentistry for Children* 34:212–218 (1967).

Cumming, B.R., and Löe, H. Consistency of plaque distribution in individuals without special home care instruction. *Journal for Periodontal Research* 8:94–100 (1973).

Davison, G.C., and Neale, J.M. *Abnormal Psychology.* New York: John Wiley and Sons, 1982.

Devine, V., Adelson, R., Goldstein, J., Valins, S., and Davison, G.C. Controlled test of the analgesic and relaxant properties of nitrous oxide. *Journal for Dental Research* 53:486–490 (1979).

Dionne, R.A., Wirdzek, P.R., Fox, P.C., and Dubner, R. Suppression of postoperative pain by the combination and nonsteroidal anti-inflammatory drug, florbiprofen and a long acting local anesthetic, etidocaine. *Journal of the American Dental Association* 108:598–601 (1984).

Duke, M.P., and Cohen, B. Locus of control as an indication of patient cooperation. *Journal of the American College of Dentistry* 41:174–178 (1974).

Egbert, L.D., Battit, G.E., Welch, C.E., and Bartlett, M.K. Reduction of post-operative pain by encouragement and instruction of patients. *New England Journal of Medicine* 270:825–827 (1964).

Elliott, R. Tonic heart rate: experiments in the effects of collative variables lead to a hypothesis about its motivational significance. *Journal of Personality and Social Psychology* 12:211–228 (1969).

Ellis, A. *A New Guide to Rational Living.* North Hollywood, CA: Wilshire Books, 1975.

Emmertsen, E. The treatment of children under general analgesia. *Journal of Dentistry for Children* 32:123–124 (1965).

Evans, R.I. Motivating changes in oral hygiene behavior: some social psychological perspectives. *Journal of Preventive Dentistry* 5:14–19 (1978).

Fink, M., Taylor, M.A., and Volavka, J. Anxiety precipitated by lactate. *New England Journal of Medicine* 281:1429 (1969).

Fisher, G.C. Management of fear in the child patient. *Journal of the American Dental Association* 57:792–795 (1958).

Folkman, S., and Lazarus, R.S. Coping in an adequately functioning middle aged population. *Journal of Health and Social Behavior* 21:219–239 (1980).

Fordyce, W.E. *Behavioral Methods for Chronic Pain and Illness.* St. Louis: C.V. Mosby, 1976.

Forehand, R.L., and McMahon, R.J. *Helping the Noncompliant Child.* New York: The Guilford Press, 1981.

Forgione, A.G., and Clark, R.E. Comments on an empirical study of the cause of dental fears. *Journal of Dental Research* 53:496 (1974).

Frankl, S.N., Fogels, H.R., and Shiere, F.R. Should the parent remain with the child in the dental operatory? *Journal of Dentistry for Children* 29:150–163 (1962).

Freidson, E., and Feldman, J.J. The public looks at dental care. *Journal of the American Dental Association* 57:325–335 (1958).

Gale, E. Fears of the dental situation. *Journal of Dental Research* 51:964–966 (1972).

Gale, E.N., and Ayer, W.A. Treatment of dental phobias. *Journal of the American Dental Association* 78:1304–1307 (1969).

Gardner, W.J., and Licklider, J.C.R. Auditory analgesia in dental operations. *Journal of the American Dental Association* 59:1144–1149 (1959).

Gardner, W.J., Licklider, J.C.R., and Weisz, A.Z. Suppression of pain by sound. *Science* 132:32–33 (1960).

Geer, J.H., Davison, G.C., and Gatchel, R.I. Reduction of stress in humans through nonveridical perceived control of aversive stimulation. *Journal of Personality and Social Psychology* 16:731–738 (1970).

George, J.M., Scott, D.S., Turner, S.P., and Gregg, J.M. The effects of psychological factors and physical trauma on recovery from oral surgery. *Journal of Behavioral Medicine* 3:291–300 (1980).

Glennon, B., and Weisz, J.R. An observational approach to the assessment of anxiety in young children. *Journal of Consulting and Clinical Psychology* 46:1246–1257 (1978).

Gold, S.L. Establishing motivating relations in preventive dentistry. *Journal of the American Society of Preventive Dentistry* 4:17–25 (1974).

Hain, J.D., Butcher, H.G., and Stevenson, I. Systematic desensitization therapy: an analysis of results in twenty-seven patients. *British Journal of Psychiatry* 112:297–307 (1966).

Hall, N., and Edmonson, H.D. The aetiology and psychology of dental fear. *British Dental Journal* 154:247–252 (1983).

Hawley, B.P., McCorkle, A.D., Wittemann, J.K., and Ostenberg, P.V. The first dental visit for children from low socioeconomic families. *Journal of Dentistry for Children* 41:376–381 (1974).

Hilgard, E.R. A neodissociation interpretation of pain reduction in hypnosis. *Psychological Review* 80:396–411 (1973).

Hirschman, R. Physiological feedback and stress reduction. In B. Ingersoll (chair), "Behavioral Approaches to Dental Fear, Pain and Stress." Symposium presented at the meeting of Society of Behavioral Medicine, New York, 1980.

Hirschman, R., Young, D., and Nelson, C. Psychologically based techniques for stress reduction. In B.D. Ingersoll and W.R. McCutcheon (Eds.), *Clinical Research in Behavioral Dentistry: Proceedings of the Second Na-*

tional Conference on Behavioral Dentistry. Morgantown, West Virginia, West Virginia University, 1979.

Hodgson, R., and Rachman, S. Disynchrony measures of fear. *Behavioral Research and Therapy* 12:319–326 (1974).

Hoffman, J.W., Benson, H., Arns, P.A., Stainbrook, G.L., Landsberg, G.L., Young, J.B., and Gill, A. Reduced sympathetic nervous system responsivity associated with the relaxation response. *Science* 215:190–192 (1981).

Hogue, D., Ternisky, M., and Iranpour, B. The responses to nitrous oxide analgesia in children. *Journal of Dentistry for Children* 38:129–133 (1971).

Hollister, L.E. *Clinical Use of Psychotherapeutic Drugs.* Springfield, Ill.: Charles C. Thomas, 1973.

Houston, B.K. Control over stress, locus of control and response to stress. *Journal of Personality and Social Psychology* 21:249–255 (1972).

Howit, J.W., and Stricker, G. Child patient response to various dental procedures. *Journal of the American Dental Association* 70:70–74 (1965).

Ireland, R.L. Introducing the child to dentistry. *Journal of the American Dental Association* 30:280–286 (1943).

Jackson, E. Patients' perceptions of dentistry. In P. Weinstein (Ed.), *Advances in Behavioral Research in Dentistry.* Seattle: University of Washington, 1978.

Janis, I.L. *Psychological Stress.* New York: Academic Press Inc., 1974, p. 284.

Jenks, L. How the dentist's behavior can influence the child's behavior. *Journal of Dentistry for Children* 31:358–366 (1964).

John, R., and Baldwin, D.C. Maternal anxiety and child behavior. *Journal of Dentistry for Children* 36:87–92 (1969).

Johnson, J.E., Levanthal, H., and Dabbs, J.M., Jr. Contribution of emotional and instrumental response processes in adaption to surgery. *Journal of Personality and Social Psychology* 20:55–64 (1971).

Johnson, R., and Baldwin, D.C. Relationship of maternal anxiety to behavior of young children undergoing dental extractions. *Journal of Dental Research* 47:801–805 (1968).

Kanfer, F.H., and Goldfoot, D.A. Self-control and tolerance of noxious stimulation, *Psychological Reports* 18:79–85 (1966).

Kardachi, B.J., and Clarke, N.G. The use of biofeedback to control bruxism. *Journal of Periodontology* 48:639–642 (1977).

Kaufman, E., Weinstein, P., and Milgrom, P. Difficulties in achieving local anesthesia: a review. *Journal of the American Dental Association* 108: 205–208 (1984).

Kazdin, A.E., and Wilcoxon, L.A. Systematic desensitization and nonspecific treatment effects: A methodological evaluation. *Psychological Bulletin* 83:729–758 (1976).

Kenney, E.B., Saxe, S.R., Lenox, J.A., Cooper, T.M., Caudill, J.S., Collins, A.R., and Kaplan, A. The relationship of manual dexterity and knowledge to performance of oral hygiene. *Journal of Periodontal Research* 11(2):67–73 (1976).

Kleber, C., Putt, M.S., and Muhler, J.C. Duration and pattern of toothbrushing in children using a gel or paste dentifrice. *Journal of the American Dental Association* 103(5):723–726 (1981).

Kleinknecht, R.A., and Bernstein, D.A. Assessment of dental fear. *Behavior Therapy,* 9:626–634 (1978).

Kleinknecht, R.A., Klepac, R.K., and Alexander, L.D. Origins and characteristics of fear of dentistry. *Journal of the American Dental Association* 86:842–848 (1973).

Kleinknecht, R.A., McGlynn, F.D., Thorndike, R.M., and Harkavy, J. Factor analysis of the Dental Fear Survey with cross validation. *Journal of the American Dental Association* 108:59–61 (1984).

Klepec, R.K. Successful treatment of avoidance of dentistry by desensitization or by increasing pain tolerance. *Journal of Behavioral Therapy and Experimental Psychology* 6:307–312 (1975).

Klorman, R., Michael, R., Hilpert, P.L., and Sveen, O.B. A further assessment of predictors of the child's behavior in dental treatment. *Journal of Dental Research,* 58:2338–2343 (1979).

Klorman, R., Ratner, J., Arata, C.L., King, J.B., Jr., and Sveen, O.B. Predicting the child's uncooperativeness in dental treatment from maternal traits, state and dental anxiety. *Journal of Dentistry for Children* 45:62–67 (1978).

Korsch, B., and Aley, E. Pediatric interviewing techniques. *Current Problems in Pediatrics* 3:1–42 (1973).

Kraper, D.C. "Some behavioral topics related to dentistry, speech and audiology." Presented at Conference of Joint Committee for Dentistry and Speech Pathology-Audiology, Ann Arbor, Michigan, March 6, 1970.

Kuno, Y. *Human Perspiration.* Springfield, IL: Thomas, 1956.

Langa, H. *Relative Analgesia in Dental Practice.* Philadelphia: Saunders, 1968.

Langer, E.J., Janis, L.L., and Wolfer, J.A. Reduction of psychological stress in surgical patients. *Journal of Experimental and Social Psychology* 11:155–165 (1975).

Laufer, D., Chosack, A., and Rosenzweig, K.A. Explanation as a means of reducing fear of dental procedures in children. *Alpha Omegan* 57:130–133 (1964).

Lautch, H. Dental phobia. *British Journal of Psychiatry* 119:151–158 (1971).

Lazarus, R.S. Some principles of psychological stress and their relation to dentistry. *Journal of Dental Research* 45:1620–1626 (1966).

Lazarus, R.S. The stress and coping paradigm. In C. Eisdorfer, D. Cohen, A. Kleinman, and P. Maxim (Eds.), *Models for Clinical Psychopathology.* Jamaica, New York: Spectrum Publications, 1981.

Lechner, V., and Wright, G.Z. Non-pharmacotherapeutic approaches to behavior management of the child patient. In G.Z. Wright (Ed.), *Behavior Management in Dentistry for Children.* Philadelphia: W.B. Saunders, 1975.

Levitas, T.C. Hand over mouth exercise. *Journal of Dentistry for Children* 19:178–182 (1974).

Lewis, T.M., and Law, D.B. Investigation of certain autonomic responses of children to specific dental stress. *Journal of the American Dental Association* 57:769–777 (1958).

Lick, J., and Bootzin, R. Expectancy factors in the treatment of fear: methodological and theoretical issues. *Psychological Bulletin* 82:917–931 (1975).

Longo, D.J. A psychophysiological comparison of three relaxation techniques and some implications for testing cardiovascular syndromes. *Social and Behavioral Medicine Abstracts,* #All, 10 (1984).

Macgreggor, I.D., and Rugg–Gunn, A.J. Survey of toothbrushing duration in 85 uninstructed English school children. *Community Dentistry and Oral Epidemiology* 7:297–298 (1979).

Machen, J.B., and Johnson, R. Desensitization, model learning, and the dental behavior of children. *Journal of Dental Research* 53:83–87 (1974).

Marks, I. *Fears and Phobias.* New York: Academic Press, 1969.

Martin, R.B., Shaw, M.A., and Taylor, P.P. The influence of prior surgical experience on the child's behavior at the initial dental visit. *Journal of Dentistry for Children* 44:443–447 (1977).

Mason, R.C., Clark, G., Reeves, R.B., and Wagner, S.B. Acceptance and healing. *Journal of Religion and Health* 8:123–142 (1969).

Mathews, A. Fear-reduction research and clinical phobia. *Psychological Bulletin* 85:390–404 (1978).

Mayo, R.W. Child management in the dental office. *Journal of Dentistry for Children* 12:48–49 (1945).

Melamed, B.G., Bennett. C., Hill, C.J., and Ronk, S. Strategies for patient management in pediatric dentistry. In B.D. Ingersoll and W.R. McCutcheon (Eds.), *Clinical research in behavioral dentistry: Proceedings of the second national conference on behavioral dentistry.* Morgantown, West Virginia, West Virginia University, 1979.

Melamed, B.G., Weinstein, D., Hawes, R., and Katin-Borland, M. Reduction of fear-related dental management problems with use of filmed modeling. *Journal of the American Dental Association* 90:822–826a (1975).

Melamed, B.G., Yurcheson, R., Fleece, E.L., Hutcherson, S., and Hawes, R. Effects of film modeling on the reduction of anxiety-related behaviors in individuals varying in level of previous experience in the stress situation. *Journal of Consulting and Clinical Psychology* 46:1357–1367 (1978).

Melzack, R. *The Puzzle of Pain,* New York: Basic Books, 1973.

Melzack, R., Guit, E.S., and Gonshor, A. Relief of dental pain by ice massage of the hand. *Canadian Medical Association Journal* 122:189–191 (1980).

Melzack, R., Weisz, A.Z., and Sprague, L.T. Strategies for controlling pain: Contributions of auditory stimulation and suggestion. *Experimental Neurology* 8:239–247 (1963).

Milgrom, P., Weinstein, P., and Kaufman, E. Student difficulties in achieving local anesthesia. *Journal of Dental Education.* 48(3):168–70 (1984).

Miller, N., and Dollard, J. *Personality and Psychotherapy.* New York: McGraw-Hill, 1950.

Miller, N.E. Learning of visceral and glandular response. *Science* 103:434–445 (1969).

Miller, S.M. Controllability and human stress: Method, evidence and theory. *Behavioral Research and Therapy* 17:287–304 (1979).

Molin, C., and Seeman, K. Disproportionate dental anxiety: clinical and nosological considerations. *Acta Odontologica Scandinavia* 28:197–212 (1979).

Moore, P.A., and Dunsky, J.L. Bupivacaine anesthesia—A clinical trial for endodontic therapy. *Oral Surgery* 55(2):176–179 (1984).

Moretti, R.J., Curtiss, G., and Hoerman, K.C. Dentist non-verbal communication skills, patient anxiety and patient treatment satisfaction. *Journal of Dental Research* 61:264 (1982).

Mussellman, R., and McClure, D. In G. Z. Wright (Ed.), *Behavioral Management in Dentistry for Children*. Philadelphia: Saunders, 1975.

Nash, D.A., Ingersoll, B.D., and Gamber, C. Contingent audiotaped reinforcement with pediatric dental patients. *Journal of Dental Research* 63:272 (1984).

Nathan, J. Assessment of anxious pedodontic patients to nitrous oxide. *Journal of Dental Research* 61:224 (1982).

Nathan, J.E. Nitrous oxide and the management of fear and anxiety in children. In R. Moretti and W.A. Ayer (Eds.), *The President's Conference of the Dentist-Patient Relationship and the Management of Fear, Anxiety and Pain,* Chicago, Ill.: American Dental Association, 1983.

Neiburger, E.J. Child response to suggestion. *Journal of Dentistry for Children* 45:396–402 (1978).

Nikias, M. Compliance with preventive oral home care regimens. *Journal of Dental Research* 59:2216–2225 (1980).

Oliver, C., and Hirschman, R. Voluntary heart rate control and perceived affects. *Journal of Dental Research* 61:8–10 (1982).

Papermaster, A.A. A psychological study of the dental patient. *Northwest Dentistry* 50:149–154 (1971).

Persson, G. General side-effects of local dental anesthesia. *Acta Odontologica Scandinavia* 27 (supplement): 53 (1969).

Pollack, S. Pain control by suggestion. *Journal of Oral Medicine* 21:89–95 (1966).

Rachman, S., and Hodgson, R.I. Synchrony and disynchrony in fear and avoidance. *Behavioral Research and Therapy* 12:311–318 (1974).

Reiss, S. Pavlovian conditioning and human fear: an expectancy model. *Behavioral Therapy* 11:300–396 (1980).

Richardson, S.S., and Kleinknecht, R.A. "Expectancy effects on anxiety and self-generated cognitive strategies in high and low dental anxious females." Presented to Washington State Psychological Association Meeting, May, 1983.

Robinson, H.B. Toothbrushing habits of 405 persons. *Journal of the American Dental Association* 33:1112–1117 (1946).

Roder, R.E., Law, D., and Lewis, T. Physiological responses of dentists to the presence of a parent in the operatory. *Journal of Dentistry for Children* 28:263–270 (1961).

Rogers, C.R. *On Becoming a Person.* Boston: Houghton Mifflin, 1961.

Rosengarten, M. The behavior of the preschool child at the initial dental visit. *Journal of Dental Research* 40:373 (1961).

Rotter, J.B. Generalized expectancies for internal versus external control of reinforcement. *Psychological Monographs: General and Applied* 80, Whole no. 609 (1966).

Rouleau, J., Ladouceur, R., and Dufour, L. Pre-exposure to the first dental treatment. *Journal of Dental Research* 60:30–34 (1981).

Rugh, J. *Biofeedback in Dentistry: Research in Clinical Application.* Phoenix, Arizona: Semantodontics, 1977.

Sackett, D.L., and Haynes, R.B. *Compliance with Therapeutic Regimens.* Baltimore, Maryland: The Johns Hopkins University Press, 1976.

Sawtell, R.O., Simon, J.F., and Simeonsson, R.J. The effects of five preparatory methods upon child behavior during the first dental visit. *Journal of Dentistry for Children* 41:37–45 (1974).

Schacter, S., and Singer, J.E. Cognitive, social and psychological determinants of emotional state. *Psychological Review* 69:379–399 (1962).

Schmitt, F.E., and Wooldridge, P.J. Psychological preparation of surgical patients. *Nursing Research* 22:108–116 (1973).

Scott, D.S., and Hirschman, R. Psychological aspects of dental anxiety in adults. *Journal of the American Dental Association* 104:27–31 (1982).

Scott, D.S., Hirschman, R., and Schroder, K. Historical antecedents of dental anxiety. *Journal of the American Dental Association* 108:42–45 (1984).

Seeman, K., and Molin, C. Psychopathology, feelings of confinement and helplessness in the dental chair, and the relationship to the dentist in patients with disproportionate dental anxiety (DDA). *ACTA Psychiatrica Scandinavica* 54:81–91 (1976).

Seeman, M., and Evans, J.W. Alienation and learning in a hospital setting. *American Social Review* 27:727–782 (1962).

Seligman, M.E.P. *Helplessness: On Depression, Development and Death.* San Francisco: W.C. Freeman, 1975.

Seligman, M.E.P., Maier, S.F., and Solomon, R.L. Unpredictable and uncontrollable aversive events. In F.R. Brush (Ed.), *Aversive Conditioning and Learning.* New York: Academic Press, 1971.

Shannon, I.L., and Isbel, G.M. Stress in dental patients: effect of local anesthetic procedures. *Dental Digest* 69:459–461 (1963).

Shapiro, D.N. Reactions of children to oral surgery experience. *Journal of Dentistry for Children* 34:97–99 (1967).

Shaw, D.W., and Thoresen, C.E. Effects of modeling and desensitization in reducing dental phobia. *Journal of Counseling Psychology* 21:415–420 (1974).

Shaw, E.G., and Routh, D.K. Effect of mothers presence on children's reaction to aversive procedures. *Journal of Pediatric Psychology* 7:33–42 (1982).

Sheehan, D.V. Panic attacks and phobias. *New England Journal of Medicine* 308:156–158 (1982).

Sheehan, D.V., Ballenger, J., and Jacobsen, G. The treatment of endogenous anxiety with phobic, hysterical and hypochondriacal symptoms. *Archives of General Psychiatry* 37:51–59 (1980).

Shoben, E.M., and Borland, L. An empirical study of the etiology of dental fears. *Journal of Clinical Psychology* 10:17–174 (1954).

Smith, T., Weinstein, P., Milgrom, P., and Getz, T. An evaluation of an institution-based dental fears clinic. *Journal of Dental Research* 63:272 (1984).

Solberg, W.K., and Rugh, J.D. The use of bio-feedback devices in the treatment of bruxism. *Journal of the Sourthern California State Dental Association* 40:852–3 (1972).

Sorenson, H.W., and Roth, G.I. A case for nitrous oxide-oxygen inhalation sedation: aid in the elimination of the child's fear of the needle. *Dental Clinics of North America* 17:769–781 (1973).

Sosa, R., Kennell, J., Klaus, M., Robertson, S., and Urrutia, J. The effect of a supportive comparison on perinatal problems, length of labor, and mother-infant interaction. *New England Journal of Medicine* 303:597–600 (1980).

Spreads, C. *Breathing—the ABC's.* New York: Harper and Row, 1978.

Starkey, P.E. Training office personnel to manage children. In G.Z. Wright (Ed.), *Behavior Management in Dentistry for Children.* Philadelphia: W.B. Saunders, 1975.

Steblay, N.M., and Blaman, A.L. Reduction of fear during dental treatment through reattribution techniques. *Journal of the American Dental Association* 105:1006–1009 (1982).

Sternbach, R.A. *Pain: Psychophysiological Analysis.* New York: Academic Press, 1968.

Szasz, T.J., and Hollender, M.H. A contribution to the philosophy of medicine—the basic models of the doctor-patient relationship. *Archives of Internal Medicine* 97:585–592 (1956).

Thompson, K.F. Hypnosis in dental practice: clinical views. In M. Weisenberg (Ed.), *The Control of Pain.* New York: Psychological Dimensions, 1977.

Thompson, S.C. Will it hurt less if I can control it? Complex answer to a simple question. *Psychological Bulletin* 90:89–101 (1981).

Valins, S. Cognitive effects of false heart rate feedback. *Journal of Personality and Social Psychology* 6:400–408 (1966).

Valins, S., and Ray. A.A. Effects of Cognitive desensitization of avoidance behavior. *Journal of Personality and Social Psychology* 7:345–350 (1967).

Venham, L.L. The effect of the parent's presence on the anxiety and behavior of children receiving dental treatment. Unpublished dissertation, Ohio State University, 1971.

Venham, L.L. T.V. helps young patients relax. *Dentistry Survey* 53:98 (1977).

Venham, L.L., Murray, P., and Gaulin-Kremer, E. Child-rearing variables affecting the preschool child's response to dental stress. *Journal of Dental Research* 58:2042–2045 (1979).

Weinstein, P., Milgrom, P., Ratener, P., Read, W., and Morrison, K. Dentists' perception of the patients: Relationship to quality of care. *Journal of Public Health Dentistry.* 38:10–21 (1978).

Weinstein, P., Milgrom, P., Kaufman, K., Fiset, L., and Ramsay, D. Efficacy of local anesthesia: Patient perceptions of failure to achieve optimal anesthesia. *General Dentistry,* in press.

Weinstein, P., Domoto, P.K., and Getz, T. Difficult children: the practical experience of 145 private practitioners. *Pediatric Dentistry* 3:303–305 (1981).

Weinstein, P., Getz, T., Ratener, P., and Domoto, P. The effects of dentists' behaviors on fear-related behaviors in children. *Journal of the American Dental Association* 104:32–38 (1982).

Weinstein, P., Getz, T., Ratener, P., and Domoto, P. Behavior of dental assistants managing young children in the operatory. *Pediatric Dentistry* 5:115–120 (1983).

Weinstein, P., Domoto, P., Getz, T., and Enger, R. Reliability and validity of a measure of confidence in child management. *Journal of Dental Research* 58:(Special Issue A), 408 (1979).

Weinstein, P., Domoto, P.K., Getz, T., and Enger, R. Reliability and validity of a measure of confidence in child management. *Pediatric Dentistry* 2:7–9 (1981).

Weinstein, P., Fiset, L., and Lancaster, B.L. Long-term assessment of a behavioral approach in plaque control using a multiple baseline design: the need for relapse research. *Patient Counseling and Health Education* 5:135–140 (1984).

Weinstein, P., Getz, T., and Milgrom, P. *Oral Self-Care: Strategies for Preventive Dentistry,* Reston, Virginia: Reston Publishing Co., Inc. 1985.

Weinstein, P., Smith, T.A., and Packer, M.A. Method for evaluating patient anxiety and the interpersonal effectiveness of dental personnel: An exploratory study. *Journal of Dental Research* 50:1324–1326 (1972).

Weinstein, P., Smith, T.A., and Bartlett, R. A study of the dental student-patient relationship. *Journal of Dental Research* 52:1287–1292 (1973).

Weisenberg, M. Pain and pain control. *Psychological Bulletin* 84:1008–1044 (1977).

Weisenberg, M. Cultural and racial reactions to pain. In M. Weisenberg (Ed.), *The Control of Pain.* New York: Psychological Dimension, 1977.

Weisenberg, M., Kreindler, M.L., Schachat, R., and Werboff, J. Interpreting palmar sweat prints: Not-so-simple measure. *Journal of Psychosomatic Research* 20:1–6 (1976).

Williams, J.A., Hurst, M.K., and Stokes, T.F. Peer observation in decreasing uncooperative behavior in young dental patients. *Behavior Modification* 7:225–242 (1983).

Wolpe, J. *Psychotherapy by Reciprocal Inhibition.* Stanford, CA: Stanford University Press, 1958.

Wright, F.A.C. Relationship of children's anxiety to the potential dental health behavior. *Community Dentistry and Oral Epidemiology* 8:189–194 (1980).

Wright, G.Z. *Behavior Management in Dentistry for Children.* Philadelphia: Saunders, 1975.

Wright, G.Z. and Alpern, G.D. Variables influencing children's cooperative behavior at the first dental visit. *Journal of Dentistry for Children* 38:60–64 (1971).

Wright, G.Z., Alpern, G.D., and Leake, J.L. The modifiability of maternal anxiety as it relates to children's cooperative dental behavior. *Journal of Dentistry for Children* 40:265–271 (1973).

Wright, G.Z., and McAulay, D.J. Current premedicating trends in pedodontics. *Journal of Dentistry for Children* 55:185–187 (1973).

Wurster, C.A., Weinstein, P., and Cohen, A.J. Communication patterns in pedodontics. *Perceptual and Motor Skills* 48:159–166 (1979).

Yates, A.J. *Theory and Practice in Behavior Therapy.* New York: John Wiley and Sons, 1970.

Index